The Nurs...

A practical approach to t...
Conduct for Nurses, Midwives and Health Visitors

Acknowledgement

This book is based on articles which appeared originally in *Nursing Times* within the series entitled 'Code of Conduct'. The author and publishers thank *Nursing Times* for permission to reproduce them.

The Nurse's Code

A practical approach to the Code of Professional
Conduct for Nurses, Midwives and Health Visitors

Irene Heywood Jones

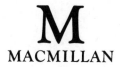

First published 1990 by
THE MACMILLAN PRESS LTD
Houndmills, Basingstoke, Hampshire RG21 2XS
and London
Companies and representatives
throughout the world

ISBN 0–333–51397–5

A catalogue record for this book is available
from the British Library.

Reprinted 1992, 1993, 1994

Printed in China

ACKNOWLEDGEMENT
The publishers would like to thank Susan Edwards for permission to use original artwork inside and on the cover of this book.

Contents

Foreword

I have long been convinced that it was essential that the ostensibly negative activity of hearings before the Professional Conduct Committee of the United Kingdom Central Council for Nursing, Midwifery and Health Visiting be turned to every possible positive advantage. Indeed, such was my view in respect of the Disciplinary Committee of the former General Nursing Council for England and Wales from a date shortly after I joined the staff of that Council in the 1970s.

The conviction that the profession should be deriving important lessons from the public consideration of the events that led to a small number of their professional peers appearing before the Committees with their professional careers at risk, led me to encourage practitioners to attend and observe hearings of cases of alleged misconduct and to write case studies about such hearings. The fact that all such case studies have been headed 'Could this happen where you work?' has emphasised my conviction that each individual case provides lessons that can be applied to many care settings.

I was therefore delighted when first approached by the author of this book and Martin Vousden of *Nursing Times* with a view to that journal using a number of my case studies in a rewritten form to inform members of the profession further and stimulate them to think about important questions of conduct and accountability.

I have been impressed with the way in which the author, applying her skills as a writer of fiction and as a teacher of nursing, has taken these case studies and presented them in a form which greatly assists personal identification with the problems experienced by the persons involved as complainants, respondents or witnesses. I have been impressed as I move around the country at the degree to which publication of these case studies – fiction but firmly based on fact – in *Nursing Times* has stimulated debate and discussion amongst many members of the profession.

I am therefore pleased to be identified with this book which presents a basic explanation of the procedures the law prescribes for the profession's regulatory body to deal with allegations of misconduct against nurses, midwives and health visitors and presents the case studies in collective form for the convenience of those who choose to use them for individual study or shared discussion. I see this as a natural extension of my desire that the matters considered by the Professional Conduct Committee be used as important learning material.

R. H. Pyne
Assistant Registrar Standards and Ethics
United Kingdom Central Council for Nursing, Midwifery and Health Visiting

Notes on contributors

Harriet Gaze
is a freelance writer and former news editor for *Nursing Times*

Irene Heywood Jones SRN, RMN, ONC, DipN, RNT
is a freelance writer and nurse tutor

Derek McCarthy RMN, SRN
is chief nurse for psychiatric services for Portsmouth District
Health Authority

Isobel Morrison MSc, BA, EN
is an enrolled nurse who, as a member of the UKCC, often sits
on the Professional Conduct Committee

Mark Scrivenger
was principal solicitor at the RCN and is now in private practice

Martin Vousden RMN
was mental health editor of *Nursing Times*

Throughout this book the terms 'nurse' and 'practitioner', used
for clarity, are interchangeable with nurse, midwife and health
visitor at all times.

Preface

Between the covers of a slim red leaflet lies information that is fundamental to the working life of every qualified nurse, mid-wife and health visitor – and to those being prepared through training. The essence of the professional role and guidance on conduct is contained on the two pages of the Code of Professional Conduct.

It is not a lot to read, especially considering the importance of the document. But the Code is still not as widely known to nurses as it should be – it is crucial for their own personal advantage, and for the benefit of the profession as a whole.

Official documents rarely make inviting or attractive reading. The information may be hard to comprehend if you have difficulty applying it to your specific area of concern and are struggling to find some personal significance.

The Code is specific in its themes of guidance, yet couched in general terms, simply because these must be interpreted in the context of prevailing circumstances. Yet some nurses find this vague and search for some tangible relevance.

The yawning gap between theory and practical application is by no means a new concept in nursing! So there was a precise intention to 'bring the Code to life', by presenting for nurses true to life scenarios with which they could identify.

This idea sparked the original 'Code of Conduct' series which first appeared in *Nursing Times* and forms the basis of this book.

The stories are based on the skeleton facts derived from actual cases appearing before the Professional Conduct Committee, with fictional details to set the scene and intensify the drama-tisation. This makes it easier for readers to envisage the circum-stances of the situation, to empathise and to try their hand at peer judgement.

The stories can be a useful learning aid, either individually or for groups, and 'Think Points' are added to suggest relevant discussion areas. Although a story is based in one particular nursing environment, the principles of conduct and performance will obviously be appropriate throughout the whole range of the profession. Quite deliberately, some of the 'Think Points' have been generalised in order to allow topics to be transferred for consideration in other areas of care.

It is all too easy to gloat at other people's misfortune and take a vicarious interest. However, the object is to encourage nurses to take a closer look at their own performance and, perhaps, to learn – or be warned – by others' mistakes. Without doubt, we should feel privileged for the opportunity to stand in someone else's shoes, to play out the exercise in a secure setting and throw around ideas and opinions among our colleagues.

Additional sections, by valued and expert contributors, give wider explanation about the organisation surrounding the subject of the book, as well as the personal experiences of people who have been involved.

Here is a safe way to examine your own conduct, your own attitudes, your own field of care, your sphere of responsibility, your interaction with colleagues and your knowledge of the profession. Discussion with colleagues will be valuable and will generate interest and understanding of the Code of Professional Conduct.

Perhaps some of the findings of the Professional Conduct Committee may surprise you. Certainly one mistake amid an unblemished history will not necessarily result in removal from the Register. Likewise, misconduct does not have to involve anything going wrong. Here is a unique opportunity to be the decision-maker and to realise what a tremendously difficult task it can be.

You are reminded that, by law, the Professional Conduct Committee hearings are open to the public and so any nurse is entitled to attend to observe cases in progress. They are held in a number of venues throughout the United Kingdom and attendance provides a most informative and salutary experience.

Nurses who have already used some of these stories have found them a helpful and enlightening learning tool and I hope they continue to stimulate discussion within the profession.

Irene Heywood Jones

1

The Policy

Why a Code of Professional Conduct?

For any nurse reading the cases which come before the Professional Conduct Committee of the UKCC, the most disquieting feature is the awful ring of familiarity.

It could happen to you

Do you recognise yourself or your colleagues in the three short accounts which follow? Each of these nurses was accused of professional misconduct in a situation which might happen at any time to any one of us. Would you have behaved any differently?

"I loved working with mentally handicapped patients but my enthusiasm was sorely tested in my new job. We were always short staffed and the regimented routines of feeding, dressing and toiletting left no time for individual care for our 24 residents. The staff were apathetic and sister showed no interest in or support for anyone who tried to offer the patients more than the bare minimum of basic care – quite the opposite in fact.

Each day was the same – an undignified, impersonal rush – and the patients had no interests and nothing to look forward to. It was very demoralising for them and for me. One patient, Angela, worried me particularly. She showed no interest in anything and seemed to have given up.

One day, when the staff nurse on duty with me had gone to tea and I was preparing a drink for Angela, a rather aggressive patient came up and kicked, slapped and spat at me. I knew I must just stand still and take it.

But when I saw that his next attack was to be on Angela my self control snapped. As he raised his leg to kick her I hit him hard on the thigh.

Afterwards I was horrified at what I had done and, after some troubled nights, confessed to the nursing officer."

"Like many district nurses I had a Crown car which I used for private motoring, paying a fee and mileage charge each month. The form filling was tedious but I did it by the book, checking the mileometer daily and keeping a careful note of my private mileage.

But last summer we were unexpectedly stretched and my caseload was even heavier than usual. My diary showed all my calls, though not necessarily in the order I made them, as timed calls and appointments took priority.

I drove hither and thither, fitting my shopping and other personal errands in during my lunch break, though my busy days left little enough time for private motoring.

In all the rushing about my paperwork got behind and I lost the habit of logging my mileage daily, only to find at the end of the month that I had to complete my travel return by referring to my diary. I worked out the mileage without looking at the mileometer and continued this practice – which saved me so much time and trouble – in the months that followed.

But when the car went in for repair in December the travel officer noticed a discrepancy of 1500 miles between the mileometer reading and my latest travel claim form."

"Everyone told me how adaptable I was, working as an enrolled nurse in the elderly medical unit. I had to be – sometimes I was the most senior nurse on duty and in charge of the ward; at other times I was relegated to dogsbody.

I enjoyed the responsibility when I was given it and did my best to get everything right. But I was not familiar with the routine of drug administration and documentation and unfortunately I made a couple of mistakes – not in themselves life threatening and not entirely my fault.

After the first mistake the nursing officer reminded me of my enrolled nurse status, and after the second she warned me formally and said that for four weeks I was to administer drugs only under the supervision of a registered nurse. But I was still often left in charge of the ward and holding the drug keys.

Just four days before the end of the suspension period, when I was in charge with a student, an auxiliary and an agency EN to help me, I telephoned Sister to come to supervise the drug round.

She came, though very busy, and duly checked and signed. In the middle of the round Mr Holloway had to rush to the toilet so although his pills were dispensed and charted they were left on the trolley. At the end of the round I cleared the trolley and locked up quickly to allow Sister to leave. Then I realised I had thrown Mr Holloway's pills into the washing up. I could not bring myself to interrupt Sister again so I asked the student to check Mr Holloway's drugs with me. She noticed that according to the chart he had already had his medication."

To discover what happened to these three practitioners you will have to read the full accounts of their cases further on in this book.

But the point is clear. There is a very thin line between acceptable behaviour and professional misconduct. Very few of us have no minor indiscretions on our consciences, even if nothing ever came of them –

nobody found out, nobody complained and, probably of greatest significance, nothing went wrong – on that occasion.

Who among us can fail to recognise ourselves in some of these stories, albeit in a modified form? 'A night break taken as a cat-nap in the empty bed in the side-room, a few celebratory beers at lunchtime, the frustrated mutterings about a difficult patient, the speedy 'routine' checking of an identification bracelet or drug sheet – do they constitute acceptable behaviour or might they verge on professional misconduct?'

But a small misdemeanour can so easily spill over to become a charge of neglecting your duty, failing in your professional responsibility. These are the kinds of situation the Code of Conduct is intended to help resolve.

Professions which form the backbone of our civilised society have earned the respect of the public, who feel confident that they can depend on the sound judgement and integrity of their members.

It is sickening, indeed frightening, to hear of people abusing the privilege and responsibility that has been bestowed by their professional standing, often using it as a guise of respectability: the racist teacher, the bullying policeman, the bribed solicitor, the molesting doctor, the thieving nurse.

Nothing is more iniquitous than corrupt professionals taking advantage of vulnerable clients. We freely hand over parts of our lives to people we trust to be upright, honest, professional in their behaviour and competent in the execution of their duty.

To ensure that the consumer is being served correctly and the good name of the profession upheld, each profession issues its own set of standards and guidelines on conduct for its practitioners. Those admitted to the body of the profession will have received an authorised training, passed some kind of assessment to qualify and be expected to conform to the code.

It is the hallmark of credibility for a profession that it is self regulating, and that those in receipt of a service have access to the organising body and recourse to an authoritative complaints procedure. And so each profession provides machinery to examine individual conduct and competence, should this be subject to question.

For nurses, the guidelines are embodied in the Code of Professional Conduct for Nurses, Midwives and Health Visitors issued by the UKCC (see pages 14–15). It is the personal responsibility of every practitioner to conform to the Code and those who are accused of violating it are subject to investigation by their peers, in order to protect public safety.

3

Daily, patients willingly and confidently accept pills, injections and treatments, sink into the oblivion of anaesthesia and sleep at night, believing their welfare, property and confidences to be in safe hands. Relatives assign responsibility for their loved ones, assured that they can rely on good care, respect and ethical practice for those not in a position to help themselves or to speak out.

There is no room for complacency. No one can afford to take risks or be off their guard, for too much is at stake.

- Lives are at stake and patients deserve to be protected from inept, incompetent or unprofessional care.
- The reputation of nursing is at stake, for the credibility of the corporate profession is reflected through individual deeds, and responses from the consumer.
- Careers are at stake. Any nurse who has been through a committee hearing, whether finally proved guilty of misconduct or not, will verify that it is a traumatic, harrowing experience. The Professional Conduct Committee has the authority to remove a nurse from the professional Register; that nurse then loses the right to practise with immediate effect.

Of course, every story has two sides. In their defence, accused nurses may offer a selection of mitigating circumstances which, whether plausible excuse or valid reason, also cover some well explored territory: overworked, understaffed, moonlighting, personality clashes, staff rivalry, communication errors, stress, burnout, personal problems.

There is no easy answer to the enquiries, no watertight system where there are so many grey areas. Cases throw up an enormous number of dilemmas. Judgement relies upon interpretation by those appointed to make a fair decision, taking account of all the circumstances and the evidence of witnesses and written records.

It is, however, a very rare case in which the only person with something to answer for is the respondent before the Committee. The pointing finger often highlights failures and inadequacies within the system.

Taking a more positive view of the Professional Conduct Committee proceedings, there may frequently be a beneficial outcome. An independent, constructive comment from the UKCC may be drawn to the attention of the managers, the relevant Health Authority or Government minister, all of

4

whom are in a position to make recommendations to improve the service.

The role of the UKCC

The safety of the public is protected by law, to ensure that it is served by well trained, competent and conscientious practitioners of nursing.

In 1983 the newly created United Kingdom Central Council for Nursing, Midwifery and Health Visiting and the four national boards finally replaced the nine statutory and other training bodies which formerly had responsibility for the varying arms of the nursing service.

The UKCC is now the statutory registration and regulatory body for the profession through an act of Parliament, the Nurses, Midwives and Health Visitors Act of 1979. The Act states that, 'The principal functions of the Central Council shall be to establish and improve standards of training, and professional conduct.'

In practice the work of the UKCC can be summarised as:

- determining education and training policies (implemented via the four national boards at local level);
- maintaining a Register of qualified practitioners;
- advising those on the Register with the aim of improving standards of care;
- regulating professional standards through the Professional Conduct Committee, which considers complaints against practitioners;
- rehabilitation of practitioners.

It is implicit in these functions that the UKCC bears the ultimate responsibility to the public on behalf of the profession. It has a duty to protect patients and honour the contract between society and the nursing profession. The safety of the public is paramount.

Professional preparation, assessment, qualification and the continued right to practise are essential stages of a professional career. While the UKCC has the corporate accountability, it, in turn, must expect personal professional accountability from individual practitioners on its Register.

So a further section of the Act states that, 'The powers of the Council shall include that of providing, in such a manner as it thinks fit, advice for nurses, midwives and health visitors on standards of professional conduct.'

This advice is embodied in the Code of Professional Conduct (see pages 14–15), which addresses major issues concerned with performance, attitude and conduct. The Code itself does not constitute a specific law. However, it is invested with legal power when used by the UKCC and national boards to regulate the nursing profession.

The Code applies to each person on the Register, from staff nurses and enrolled nurses at the grass roots, through to educators and senior managers, with obvious regard to each practitioner's sphere of responsibility. It is not something for managers to use to make their staff toe the line but a professional guide for every practitioner.

The first paragraph of the Code encapsulates crucial elements of professional responsibility and is worth examining.

Each registered nurse, midwife and health visitor shall act, at all times, in such a manner as to justify public trust and confidence, to uphold and enhance the good standing and reputation of the profession . . . .

Nurses are public figures who are generally held in high regard. As representatives of your profession you must always consider the consequences of your actions and behaviour, both on and off duty. It is worth remembering that criminal convictions of any nature, even unrelated to your work, can affect your registration status and most will be notified to the National Board.

Each registered nurse . . . shall act, at all times, . . . to serve the interests of society.

It may seem to be stating the obvious to say the profession exists because of patients. Yet it is not unknown for some nurses, at times, to be so guided by self interest that the patient becomes almost incidental.

Throughout all the guidance, advice and statements given by the UKCC, nothing is more striking than its continued reiteration of 'the primacy of the patient'.

Each registered nurse . . . shall act . . . and above all to safeguard the interests of individual patients and clients.

And this must be, without a doubt, what the patients and their relatives expect of a trained nurse providing professional care.

6

The subsequent 14 parts of the Code, together with the vital stem which reinforces personal professional accountability, touch on important areas relevant to practice.

You may at first find it difficult to relate these generalised themes to your own sphere of practice. But it is impossible to be more specific, for the Code has to be interpreted within the context of each individual situation, involving any number of factors.

It is the aim of the case studies in this book to illustrate just how this happens in practice and to show that varying circumstances can influence the final judgement.

The UKCC has had a number of requests for greater clarification in several areas and has responded with advisory papers to accompany the Code of Professional Conduct, on *Confidentiality, Advertising, Administration of Medicines* and *Exercising Accountability*.

The professional conduct function is best summarised in extracts from an opening address in 1983 by Dame Catherine Hall, then Chairman of the UKCC.

"I believe that the professional conduct function should be seen in positive terms – as one of the means through which a regulatory body, acting on behalf of the profession, honours the contract between the profession and society by ensuring that any member of the profession who has failed to meet the trust which society has placed on him or her is not permitted to continue to practise, or, if the failure has not been a serious one, is reminded of the standard which professional practitioners are expected to meet.

It is also in the interest of the professional practitioner to be 'called to order' by fellow practitioners, if there has been a failure to maintain acceptable standards of professional competence or conduct; otherwise the individual could be exposed to further hazards with an even more serious outcome.

However, it is recognised that, in some instances, individual failures are due to ill health, rather that to culpable negligence or criminal intent. Accordingly, a separate mechanism has been set up to deal with those whose alleged professional misconduct, or whose criminal conviction, may be the effects of a health problem.

The underlying philosophy of the professional conduct function is to protect the public, to promote high standards of professional practice and conduct of nurses, midwives and health visitors, to ensure that justice is being done, and is seen to be done, in respect of those who are brought within this function and that every encouragement is given to the individual practitioner to re-establish himself or herself, if it can be demonstrated that this is not contrary to the public interest. Justice must be tempered by mercy, but sentimentality has no place in the administration of justice.

I hope in considering the means, we will all bear in mind the end – the maintenance and improvement of standards of professional conduct to befit a profession on whose competence and conduct individuals are dependent in times of their greatest vulnerability."

Who knows the Code?

by Martin Vousden

How much do you know about the Code of Professional Conduct? It has been quoted from innumerable public platforms and in many articles and books. But, without looking it up, can you say who produced the Code, in what year it first appeared and in what circumstances you cannot use your nursing qualification?

For your own interest, try to answer the questions in the following table and see how you compare with participants from a *Nursing Times* ward sisters' conference in Manchester. They answered the same questions but, unlike you, they did not have the opportunity to cheat. The penalty for looking up the Code will be instant removal of your name from the Register!

How did you get on? If you are anything like the 234 conference attenders who answered these questions, you will probably be surprised by how much you did not know.

For example, nearly a quarter wrongly believed that the Code applies to student nurses. A slightly higher percentage think it is advisory and not directive, something that must be of concern to nurse practitioners, managers and the UKCC itself.

But there were some revealing comments at the foot of the questionnaire where respondents were asked for additional views on the Code. A junior sister from Glamorgan said, 'I still feel that the Code should be explained and its implications stressed to all nurses – some still feel it is unimportant.'

Another sister, this time from Kingston and Esher, thinks the Code is, 'not widely known among staff nurses and ENs; newly qualified staff do not receive a copy.' One cry from the heart, by an anonymous respondent who claims never to have read the Code or to have had access to a copy was, 'All information is hearsay. Sorry, but we remain, as always, misinformed.'

A charge nurse in London believes the Code, 'should be the

Professional Conduct Code test

Question	Choice of answer (where given)
1 When was the Code first published?	(a) 1963 (b) 1973 (c) 1983
2 Which organisation produced the Code?	
3 To whom does the Code apply?	(a) everyone on the Register (b) registered, but not enrolled nurses (c) everyone on the Register and students in nursing
4 What status does the Code have?	(a) advisory (b) directive
5 Name one situation in which the Code advises nurses to disclose confidential information.	
6 What does the Code advise a nurse to do if she/he believes standards of care to be inadequate?	
7 Name the areas covered by any or all of the four documents which have been produced to expand on different aspects of the Code.	
8 What does the Code say is the primary duty of nurse, midwife or health visitor?	(a) to uphold the good standards and reputation of the profession (b) to take every reasonable opportunity to maintain and improve professional knowledge and competence (c) to safeguard the interests of individual patients and clients
9 Name one situation in which the Code advises nurses not to use their nursing qualification.	
10 Have you ever read the Code?	(a) yes (b) no
11 Do you own or have access to a copy of the Code?	

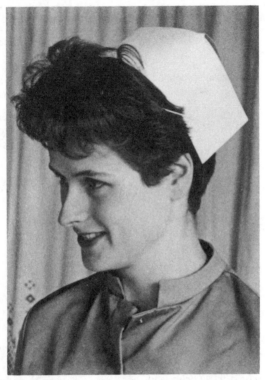

final arbiter for the nurse and her conduct where nursing and general management are in conflict.' And one respondent, who obviously believes that discretion is the better part of valour, answered the first question (wrongly), presumably glanced at the remaining questions and decided to go no further.

But the comment that best summed up the majority view came from a sister in Newham who clearly echoed the thoughts of many respondents when she said, 'I wish I'd read it better.' A footnote, obviously added later, bore the admission, 'I have just re-read the Code of Conduct and am ashamed at my lack of knowledge!'

The first question, asking when the Code was first produced, delivered in 196 (84%) correct answers identifying 1983 as the year. Nearly a tenth, 23 people (9.8%), thought the answer was 1973. A few hippy retreads remembered the Code coming out in 1963, and six people were honest enough to admit being 'don't knows'.

A slightly higher percentage (87.1%), got the second question right and knew the Code was produced by the UKCC. But 19 (8.1%), possibly harking back to fond memories of matrons and starched aprons, named the GNC as author, while eight people did not know. The RCN and ENB received one vote each.

There was less agreement on question three. Almost a quarter, 56 (23.9%), wrongly believed that students in training were governed by the Code. One hundred and sixty five respondents (70.5%), said correctly that it applied to everyone on the Register, including enrolled nurses. Eight people (3.4%) thought ENs were excluded and five (2.1%) were 'don't knows'.

There was a similar division of opinion about question four. One hundred and sixty four people (70%), correctly said the Code was directive, while 65 (27.7%) wrongly described it as advisory. Again, five people, although it is not known if they are the same five, did not know.

The 'don't knows' really came into their own in question five and comprised the second largest group of answers given. As it was a more open question, there was a wider variety of response when asked, 'According to the Code there are some situations where a nurse should disclose confidential information – can you name one such situation?'

Sixty five people (27.7%) could not. The largest group, comprising 99 people (42.3%) rightly said, 'when required by law'. No one gave the alternative correct answer of, 'when required by the order of a court' but two people (0.8%) rightly said, 'in the public interest'. Forty eight people (20.5%) thought confidential information could be disclosed if the care or well being of the patient was at risk.

Two respondents each said it should happen, 'under the Data Protection Act', 'with consent from the patient', and 'when approved by the medical staff'. This last point presumably proves there is a corner of the country where medicine still rules – OK? One vote each was given to the headings 'relating to abortion', 'drug error', 'concerning misconduct from a professional to the patient', and 'if suspended' (suspended from what?).

Question six also left a lot of room for personal comment. The correct answer is to, 'make known to appropriate persons or authorities any circumstances that could militate against safe standards of practice.'

By far the largest group, 95 people (40.5%) felt it encumbent on a nurse to report the matter to a manager or senior nurse. A further 30 (12.8%) believe this is not enough and the immediate or line manager should be circumvented in order to report to a 'higher' authority; either a general manager or the health authority. On similar lines, another 39 people (16.6%) believed the nurse should document/put in writing her unhappiness and presumably these reports would be passed up the management hierarchy in some way.

This means that, by one route or another, 164 people (70%) would inform a senior that an unacceptable standard exists. Thirty five people (14.9%) – perhaps a surprisingly large group – were 'don't knows'; 19 (8.1%) said they would take steps to improve the situation, seven (2.9%) would report direct to the UKCC and a further two (0.8%) would discuss it with someone. Other answers, receiving one endorsement each, were 'refer to ENB', 'find out why', 'challenge', 'maintain', and, conjuring up delightful images, 'expose them'.

Confused? You will be because question seven produced 26 different responses, only four of which were correct. Respondents were asked which further four documents had been produced by the UKCC, expanding on different areas of the Code (some have labelled these documents 'Son of Code I, II, III and IV').

It is not possible to give the answers in percentages because 77 respondents gave no answers, 55 gave one answer, 63 gave two and 39 gave three. This makes a total of 298 answers from 234 respondents: the logistics of putting that into percentages would baffle Einstein.

Most people, 117 in all, rightly remembered a document on the administration of drugs. A further 65 correctly mentioned confidentiality but only two recalled the first 'Son of Code' on advertising. It becomes particularly interesting to analyse the documents and reports that nurses have read, believing them to emanate from the UKCC and to be offspring of the original Code.

Nineteen mentioned a document on 'the extended role of the nurse', 11 said 'the UKCC handbook' and a further 11 said 'the Code of Professional Conduct' – presumably referring to the second, slightly modified, edition. These are the only answers to get into double figures but other respondents, ranging from one to eight, thought they had seen Council documents on psychiatry, midwives/health visitors, nurses, Project 2000, ethics, research, standards of care, education, data protection, industrial action, AIDS, complaints, conscientious objectors and the disciplinary process.

The next question asked if the primary duty of the nurse, midwife or health visitor, according to the Code, was to: (a) 'uphold the good standards and reputation of the profession', (b) 'take every reasonable opportunity to maintain and improve professional knowledge and competence' or (c) 'safeguard the interest of individual patients and clients.'

One hundred and forty six people (62.3%) knew the primary duty of the nurse was to safeguard the interest of individual patients and clients. But there was a fairly equal division of opinion among the other choices. Twenty four (10.2%) plumped for answer (a), 36 (15.3%) for (b) and 28 (11.9%) were 'don't knows'.

Question nine asked respondents to name one situation in which they should not use their nursing qualification. Here, finally, the 'don't knows' were almost in the majority; perhaps proving once and for all that the meek shall inherit the earth. One hundred and thirteen people (48.2%), almost half, came into this category. The next largest group with 78 replies (33.3%) concerned advertising, the correct answer. In the words of the Code, the practitioner shall, 'avoid the use of professional qualifications in the promotion of commercial products...'.

Only one other answer got into double figures and this concerned the 14 people (5.9%) who mentioned first aid or attending road traffic accidents. This presumably reflects the fear some nurses have about being prosecuted for action they might take when off duty.

Other answers, all receiving fewer than 10 votes each, were 'when struck off the Register', 'dealing with sales reps', 'when drunk', 'to gain personal advantage', 'dealing with the press or media' and 'if standing for public office'.

Finally, respondents were asked if they had ever read the Code and if they had their own copy or had access to a copy. It is not perhaps surprising that 211 people (90.1%) claimed they had read the Code. But 16 respondents (6.8%) admitted they had not and seven (2.9%) did not answer the question, suggesting that nearly 10% of our sample had never seen the Code.

The Code of Professional Conduct
for Nurses, Midwives and Health Visitors

Each registered nurse, midwife and health visitor shall act, at all times, in such a manner as to justify public trust and confidence, to uphold and enhance the good standing and reputation of the profession, to serve the interests of society, and above all to safeguard the interests of individual patients and clients.

Each registered nurse, midwife and health visitor is accountable for his or her practice, and, in the exercise of professional accountability shall:

1 Act always in such a way as to promote and safeguard the well being and interests of patients/clients.

2 Ensure that no action or omission on his/her part or within his/her sphere of influence is detrimental to the condition or safety of patients/clients.

3 Take every reasonable opportunity to maintain and improve professional knowledge and competence.

4 Acknowledge any limitations of competence and refuse in such cases to accept delegated functions without first having received instruction in regard to those functions and having been assessed as competent.

5 Work in a collaborative and co-operative manner with other health care professionals and recognise and respect their particular contributions within the health care team.

6 Take account of the customs, values and spiritual beliefs of patients/clients.

7 Make known to an appropriate person or authority any conscientious objection which may be relevant to professional practice.

8 Avoid any abuse of the privileged relationship which exists with patients/clients and of the privileged access allowed to their property, residence or workplace.

9 Respect confidential information obtained in the course of professional practice and refrain from disclosing such information without the consent of the patient/client, or a person entitled to act on his/her behalf, except where disclosure is required by law or by the order of a court or is necessary in the public interest.

10 Have regard to the environment of care and its physical, psychological and social effects on patients/clients, and also to the adequacy of resources, and make known to appropriate persons or authorities any circumstances which could place patients/clients in jeopardy or which militate against safe standards of practice.

11 Have regard to the workload of and the pressures on professional colleagues and subordinates and take appropriate action if these are seen to be such as to constitute abuse of the individual practitioner and/or to jeopardise safe standards of practice.

12 In the context of the individual's own knowledge, experience, and sphere of authority, assist peers and subordinates to develop professional competence in accordance with their needs.

13 Refuse to accept any gift, favour or hospitality which might be interpreted as seeking to exert undue influence to obtain preferential consideration.

14 Avoid the use of professional qualifications in the promotion of commercial products in order not to compromise the independence of professional judgement on which patients/clients rely.

2

The Process

Professional Conduct Committee proceedings

Just as the Code of Conduct provides a frame of reference to guide practitioners in their professional role, it also provides a backcloth against which to judge allegations of their misconduct.

The UKCC, in its regulatory capacity, investigates complaints against practitioners on the Register. The appointed Committee of the UKCC is the only authority with the legal power to remove from the Register a practitioner, who thereby loses the right to practise.

Within the integrated system, the old style 'disciplinary committee' has become the UKCC Professional Conduct Committee which, while retaining a necessary disciplinary function to protect the vulnerable public, offers positive support, guidance and advice. It does not exist solely to mete out punishment. If at any time during an investigation it seems that there may be physical or mental problems affecting a nurse's fitness to practise, the case can be referred to the recently established Health Committee, who will also consider cases referred directly by colleagues or members of the public.

Those who are eventually removed from the Register have an opportunity to apply for restoration later.

The UKCC has a statutory responsibility to give all complaints a thorough, comprehensive investigation, to ensure the complainant has his or her case fully heard and that the respondent is allowed a proper defence. Nurses are judged by other nurses, a representative peer group with the necessary understanding, knowledge and experience of nursing matters.

The purposes of the Professional Conduct Committee are:

- to protect patients and the public;
- to maintain and improve standards of care;
- to rehabilitate practitioners.

Sources of complaint

Anybody from within the profession or from the lay public can bring an allegation of misconduct. If a nurse's conduct is questionable, investigation must ascertain that nurse's continued right to registration and eligibility to practise.

Professional managers

Following an incident dealt with locally, a manager may question whether the nurse concerned should practise at all, and refer the case to the UKCC.

Colleagues

Nurses who observe unacceptable behaviour by colleagues should expose the bad practice of others. This is by no means easy to do and requires considerable courage, but the Code clearly indicates a responsibility to speak out in the interests of patients.

Patients and relatives

Individuals who receive poor care are those most entitled to complain about a particular nurse. Current awareness of consumers' rights means that people are increasingly inclined to make their dissatisfactions known, but there are probably just as many, if not more, who suffer in silence. Relatives fear reprisal or recriminations towards the vulnerable patient.

Ignorance of the system also deters action, although information can be obtained from the hospital management, Community Health Council or Citizens' Advice Bureau.

Private citizens

Any member of the public can bring a complaint. Some examples might be: a visitor observing mismanagement of another patient in the ward; a neighbour encountering a district nurse; another professional person or volunteer working alongside a nurse; someone on a bus overhearing a conversation that breaches confidentiality.

Criminal courts

If a nurse is found guilty of one of a wide range of offences in a criminal court, the relevant National Board is notified of that conviction. The offence does not have to be work-related, but the Board will consider whether it has professional significance.

Some offences have more of a bearing on a professional practitioner than others.

The bodies are bound to accept guilt established in a court of law as conclusive and to act upon that verdict without query. Nurses who are advised to plead guilty or who choose not to appeal against a conviction should bear this in mind.

The kinds of offences that are commonly reported are shoplifting, failing to pay a fare on public transport, petty theft, drink or drug-related offences, driving offences, physical assault, dishonesty and indecency.

There may also be some instances when a nurse's behaviour at work will coincidentally bring criminal charges, such as theft and abuse of drugs, physical abuse or manslaughter, theft from a patient, or fraudulent use of hospital property.

National Board investigation

All complaints are first referred to a National Board Investigating Committee, which is advised by a solicitor. At this stage a decision is made on formal documentary evidence only.

The allegation is considered in the context of the situation. Evidence is gathered from the workplace on the circumstances surrounding the incident, together with some information about the practitioner's professional history.

Written statements are requested from the respondent, complainant and other witnesses but these people are not present at the meeting.

The practitioner in question is informed of the allegations or report of a conviction and invited to submit a statement. She or he is also advised of the existence of the Nurses' Welfare Service which is specifically available to offer support and advice in these matters (see page 26).

The Investigating Committee must make one of the following decisions.

- The nurse has no case to answer so the case is closed.
- No action is to be taken but the nurse is referred to the pertinent clauses of the Code of Conduct.
- The case should be referred to the Health Committee.
- The case is so serious that removal from the Register in the public interest is a distinct possibility. It is then referred to the UKCC Professional Conduct Committee.

Professional Conduct Committee hearing

Meetings are held in various parts of the United Kingdom to cover the geographical spread of cases, in order to lessen the time, expense and disruption to those involved. This also makes it possible for members of the profession and the public to observe the profession regulating itself. Whatever the location or venue, the hearing functions in a legal setting and is respected as such.

The legislation requires an open hearing, to enable the public access to observe proceedings that are held in their interest.

From the pool of 45 UKCC members, five are chosen to form the Conduct Committee, with one acting as chairman. Of the other four, at least two members will be from the same field of care as the nurse who is the subject of the hearing, for example, midwifery, psychiatry or mental handicap, if the council membership makes this possible.

An experienced legal assessor sits with the Committee to advise on matters of law and admissability of evidence but is not involved in any decision making.

This Committee does not have access to the documents previously made available to the National Board Investigating Committee. Members must make their decision on the evidence presented at this public hearing and on nothing else.

The standard of proof that the law requires is proof beyond reasonable doubt – hearsay or circumstantial evidence is insufficient.

It is perhaps important to emphasise at this point the necessity for nurses always to maintain clear and accurate written records of events that occur in the course of their work. There is the possibility they may be called as legal evidence in the future. These contemporaneous records become very important in evidence.

The Council's solicitor presents the case. The practitioner usually has a representative from a professional organisation or trade union to offer the defence. A member of the Nurses' Welfare Service (see page 26) may also be present. There is cross-examination of the respondent and the evidence from witnesses, who may be compelled to attend by subpoena if necessary.

When the Committee goes *in camera*, the public and press are excluded from the deliberations. Following all the evidence the Committee will retire to discuss the case, reach a decision by vote and arrive at a judgement. It is a collective appraisal by peers. There is always the option to refer the case to the Health Committee.

The Professional Conduct Committee must initially decide whether the charges are proved and the alleged incident did occur.

- If the answer is no, then the case is closed and the file destroyed.
- If the answer is yes, it did happen, then the Committee must decide if that which was proved amounts to professional misconduct.
- If the answer is no, it is not professional misconduct, then the case is closed and the file destroyed.
- If the answer is yes, it is professional misconduct, there is a mitigation/aggravation stage.

At this point testimonials and references are heard in support of past competent performance, often gathered from colleagues and patients. There may also be a report from the Nurses' Welfare Service on the social circumstances of the practitioner. Also revealed is any proven misconduct within the preceding 10 years that did not result in removal from the Register, plus previous convictions or disciplinary action in employment.

Finally, the Committee makes a judgement from three options:

- To postpone judgement for a stated period, during which time the option for removal from the Register is kept open but the practitioner remains eligible to practise. The person concerned returns for a resumed hearing, having fulfilled the prescribed conditions, such as employers' references or treatment for drug or alcohol abuse.
- Not to remove the name from the Register, despite proven misconduct, but to give the practitioner professional advice, referring to the Code of Conduct. A record of the proven misconduct is retained for 10 years and will be produced if further misconduct is proved before a Professional Conduct Committee within that period.
- To remove the practitioner's name from the professional Register, which takes immediate effect.

Appeal machinery
Any practitioner can appeal against the decision to remove his or her name from the Register through an appeal court within

A summary of Professional Conduct investigation proceedings

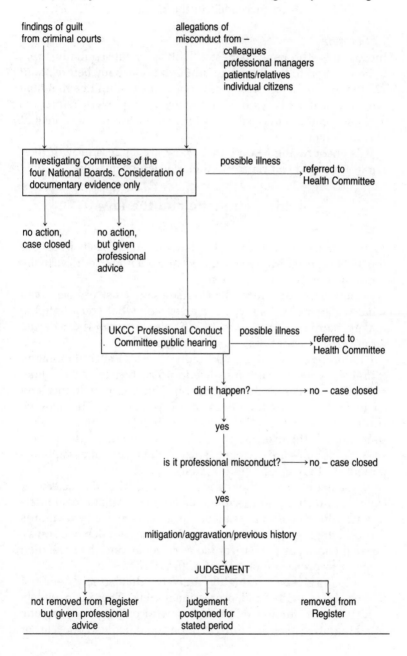

findings of guilt
from criminal courts

allegations of
misconduct from –
        colleagues
        professional managers
        patients/relatives
        individual citizens

Investigating Committees of the
four National Boards. Consideration of
documentary evidence only

possible illness   referred to
Health Committee

no action,
case closed

no action,
but given
professional
advice

UKCC Professional Conduct
Committee public hearing

possible illness   referred to
Health Committee

did it happen? ⟶ no – case closed

yes

is it professional misconduct? ⟶ no – case closed

yes

mitigation/aggravation/previous history

JUDGEMENT

not removed from Register
but given professional
advice

judgement
postponed for
stated period

removed from
Register

three months, although the removal stands during that time. There have been six cases during the UKCC's first five year term, one of which succeeded in the English High Court.

Restoration

Individuals who have been 'struck off' may subsequently apply to be restored to the Register, although not usually before about 12–18 months. They must give proof to the Committee that they are worthy of being restored, normally by employers' references and personal testimonials and by demonstrating new insight and understanding.

It is encouraging to note that many are successful with their application and can return to their chosen profession.

Ethics, etiquette and the law
by Mark Scrivenger

Many nurses seem to think the law dominates their lives, but the 1979 Nurses, Midwives and Health Visitors Act is virtually the only law there is on nursing.

Society says, in effect, 'You nurses say "trust us, we know what we are doing" so we have given you what you wanted to make it happen. Get on with it.' Who else but a nurse can decide what nursing is or what should be done?

Discussing standards and procedures raises issues of morality. Morality, when broadly translated into a practice or discipline, sets out the rules of the relationship between practitioner and client and becomes the ethics of the profession. This may be contrasted with the rules dealing with relationships between practitioners themselves, which is the etiquette of the profession. Some rules are inviolate, such as theft from or assault on a patient. Others give room for choices.

Nurses are given the freedom to organise the selection, training, practice and discipline of nursing without legal interference. But the ultimate sanction of unreasonable behaviour is through the organs of the State, such as the law. Behaviour may be so antisocial as to be regarded as criminal, and the State then steps in to prosecute on behalf of the community.

It is conceivable, if highly unlikely, that society will not tolerate a generally held professional view. There is a widely held belief in nursing that it is unlawful or illegal for anyone other than two qualified nurses, or one qualified and one learner nurse, to a do a drug round. There is no legal basis for this. If there were, a parent could not give a drug to a sick child.

Anyone can administer drugs; a domestic, the hospital gardener, the visitors or the patients themselves. The law will not prevent a drug administration policy which has the gardener giving drugs, but when the inevitable disaster occurs, a judge will savage whoever was stupid enough to introduce it.

Unqualified people handing out drugs like sweets may sooner or later kill someone. Experience and common sense – or custom and practice to use other terms – show that people who know drug dosages, likely effects and what to do if something goes wrong are safer. Curiously, the recognised procedure in which two staff check each other ought to be virtually foolproof, but produces an alarming number of mistakes. Perhaps each nurse unconsciously relies on the other and responsibility falls between them.

In law, each person is responsible for his or her own actions and their reasonable and probable consequences. Hitting someone with a car, or giving the wrong drug is the same in principle, although the harm caused will be different. In ethics, too, responsibility is measured, not in a court by lawyers investigating what a reasonably competent person would have done, but by the practitioners themselves sitting in judgement.

In nursing, the National Boards make a preliminary assessment of whether infraction of the ethical rules may have occurred. If so, the UKCC will give full consideration through the Professional Conduct Committee. If the nurse has not met acceptable standards of practice or behaviour the Committee will express concern or take appropriate action.

Guidance to practitioners about what the rules are, for both ethics and etiquette, are given through the UKCC's Code of Professional Conduct, which sets up the norms of acceptable professional behaviour. This framework is regarded as reasonable and proper by the vast majority of practitioners.

The Code has no legal standing. Guidance on ethics or etiquette is not law. Law and ethics should not be confused, any more than law and justice, although the Code could become of legal significance. For example, it is conceivable that a manager could be cross-examined about his or her knowledge of the Code's existence. Ignorance of it, admittedly unlikely, would be an admission of failure to reach the standard of an ordinary competent manager.

On the other hand, admitting its existence could produce further questioning about the meaning or value of particular paragraphs. An adversary could call further evidence about whether the manager had achieved the standards envisaged by the Code. Failure to do so would provide strong evidence of negligence.

Parliament has given nurses the power to decide what is acceptable in nursing. The Code expresses that power as a statement of acceptable standards.

It does not, however, indicate the complete scope of a practitioner's responsibility. Matters of professional misconduct may occur on duty, as they usually do, and be recognised as such by the Code. Or they may occur off duty, which may effect the general esteem of nursing in the public eye.

An act may be so antisocial as to be criminal, but it may have nothing to do with nursing. Hitting a neighbour with an axe, or theft from a local shop, is nothing to do with work, but may result in a conviction or imprisonment. All convictions are automatically reported to the relevant National Board. Part of the trade-off of being allowed to self regulate nursing is that nurses' behaviour is on public display. Most criminal convictions would be considered to be professional misconduct, but not all; some offences are worse than others.

Criminal acts may arise out of practice. Ill treating or assaulting a patient or theft from a patient or colleague are examples of more heinous acts deserving professional censure and action.

Most allegations of misconduct arise from mistakes at work. Such errors are usually mechanical, such as miscalculating a drug dosage or giving a wrong drug. Sometimes they concern judgement, such as deciding whether to take a certain course of action. Inaction as well as action can be crucial.

The law draws a distinction here which may not exist in matters of alleged misconduct. Giving the wrong drug or dosage may not harm the patient. In law there must be harm or injury suffered or there will be no claim, or one too trivial to worry about. Nevertheless, the same action could be considered to be professional misconduct. Whether the consequences of an act ought to be taken into account in cases of professional misconduct, as they are in law, is probably a matter for that most uncommon quality – especially in the health service – common sense.

Clinical nursing is the most fertile field for error, and allegations of professional misconduct. But teachers and managers are not immune. In all cases, the test is the same: whether a reasonably competent practitioner would have done the same. A tutor or clinical teacher who teaches badly may send students into the wards to cause harm to the patients or themselves. It is their responsibility to teach well.

A few cases before the Conduct Committee concerning nurse managers would crystallise the managerial mind wonderfully. The clinical nurse's duty is to the patient and the teacher's to the student. Managers have a wider duty. The consequences of their getting it wrong can be more far-reaching.

The Code recognises this, particularly in paragraphs 10 and 11. Under paragraph 10, the manager has to consider the resources to provide a proper and safe standard of practice for the patients. Paragraph 11 is concerned with the duty to consider the workload and pressures on staff which will enable them, ultimately, to carry out the safe practices described in paragraph 10.

This is fine in theory, but resources cost money that managers do not have, although it is no defence in law to claim lack of money. The manager's function is not to find money, but to ensure patients and staff are properly looked after.

Accordingly, staff shortages, inadequate training, equipment or resources may lead to successful claims of negligence based on managerial failure which caused damage to the person injured, whether patient or member of staff. The Conduct Committee may also see it as a breach of the Code, even if in law there is no case because no injury is suffered.

An inadequate policy or procedure must be corrected. A precondition of ensuring safe standards of patient care is to look after the staff. Many nurses see standards as the most important part of nursing without understanding what is needed to achieve them. Unless the conditions are right for the practitioner, standards will not be achieved or maintained. Nurses fearful about their jobs, feeling undervalued, are demoralised and cannot deliver the care they wish. This is why there are so many people leaving nursing.

Misconduct might be alleged against an off duty nurse, even where no criminal law is broken or civil action available. What if a nurse in uniform fails to stop at a motor accident? There is no legal requirement to do so. There is no such law recognised by the courts as the law of the good Samaritan. No doubt most nurses do stop and assist, but failing to do so is a matter of moral disapproval at best, not one where a legal sanction is available.

Perhaps, in refusing to be involved, a nurse would be considered to have committed misconduct even if she felt that, being off duty, it was nothing to do with her. Or, are nurses on duty 24 hours a day, as the UKCC seems to think? There is no legal ground for this view, but a profession is entitled to fix its own rules.

That nurses should take this view may reflect nursing's own uncertainty about itself and its image. But that is another story.

The Nurses' Welfare Service

It is difficult to guess how any one of us might react on learning that we face allegations of professional misconduct. Yet, for such a profound personal and professional crisis, some possibilities spring readily to mind: shock, bewilderment, despair, devastation, fear, anger, confusion, sadness, anxiety.

With the potential threat of removal from the Register and consequent loss of right to practise, questions hang over livelihood, financial commitments and future employment, especially if nursing is the only job you have ever known.

There can be the attendant blow to self esteem and confidence, status and personal identity, together with the effects on relationships with employer, colleagues and family. A huge cloud overshadows career prospects.

This is not a life event to be underestimated, and the whole stressful experience, whatever the outcome, can be extremely worrying and upsetting. Needless to say it is not an easy time to struggle alone with unfamiliar official documentation and procedures.

Luckily the Nurses' Welfare Service, a social work agency, offers support, both practical and personal. It is a charitable organisation, administered by the Nurses' Welfare Trust. Although it has a close working relationship with the statutory bodies, it operates separately and independently.

The service is free, voluntary and strictly confidential, offering information, advice, guidance and counselling to practitioners whose conduct is being questioned by the statutory bodies.

A practitioner is initially informed by the relevant National Board of the allegation of misconduct or notification of a court conviction, and is invited to submit a statement for consideration by the Investigating Committee. At the same time he or she is told of the existence of the Nurses' Welfare Service and the help it is able to provide.

The service complements the work of the staff organisations and is of immense benefit for those without other representation.

It is obviously very useful to have access to an impartial welfare officer, with whom to discuss the events and problems surrounding the allegations. The officer can also help the nurse to understand the purpose of the investigation and the machinery that exists at various levels for Conduct Committee proceedings and the options available.

The nurse can be helped to prepare the statement for the National Board Investigating Committee. Counselling is given as appropriate, to enable the nurse to plan ahead realistically.

Should the case be referred to the UKCC Professional Conduct Committee, the welfare officer can provide ongoing support and reassurance during the intervening waiting period, which is often unavoidably prolonged. The practitioner may already have been through a local disciplinary procedure and be suspended from work. It can cause considerable strain to live such a limbo existence with your fate hanging over you.

The welfare officer can provide further support by accompanying and representing the practitioner at the hearing.

With the consent of the nurse, the welfare officer can make a social background report, which aims to provide a comprehensive, objective and honest appraisal of the nurse's personal and professional circumstances. This can assist the relevant committee to view the matter under investigation in context, and would be presented at the mitigation stage of the PCC.

If a nurse loses the right to practise, he or she must face up to a future as a non-nurse. This presents a difficult, painful period of readjustment. Employment prospects can be limited, especially if a criminal offence was involved.

Some nurses want to continue working in the caring field and many opt for jobs as auxiliary nurses or care assistants. This obviously does provide valuable experience that may be looked upon favourably by the committee which considers restoration to the Register. However it is not without its problems and could put the practitioner in an invidious situation if she is tempted, or indeed expected, to act out of role and utilise her knowledge as a qualified nurse.

Long term counselling may be required in the rehabilitation period for those intending to aim for restoration to the Register.

At whatever point a practitioner decides to elicit the help of the Nurses' Welfare Service, he or she must be relieved and gratefully reassured that a service can provide information, understanding and support that is specific to his or her need.

It is an enlightened profession that can lend a caring hand for the carer in trouble and work positively towards rehabilitation of practitioners.

3

The People

Respondents

When nightmare becomes reality

by Martin Vousden

Most nurses who read of colleagues being charged with errors in drug administration will have thought, 'There but for the grace of God go I.' It seems that making a mistake while administering medicines is the sort of thing that almost all nurses have done, or believe themselves capable of doing.

For Pauline Farrell, two such errors completely changed her life and led to her admission to a psychiatric hospital; an experience which, along with an appearance in front of the UKCC Professional Conduct Committee, she will never forget.

Her problems began when she was on night duty with a student nurse and the wrong drug was given to a patient, either by Ms Farrell or the student; she cannot remember which. The reason for her vagueness is that she simply cannot recall the incident. The student nurse did not report it for nearly two months, by which time Ms Farrell had difficulty remembering the night in question. The student waited so long because initially she decided not to report the incident but seven weeks later she attended a lecture which emphasised the importance of always reporting such situations and realised she had been wrong not to approach senior staff earlier.

Ms Farrell remembers being angry with the student for waiting so long to make a complaint and also felt anger towards her employers who, after a hearing, gave her a formal written warning.

'I thought this was very unfair,' she said, 'because I had been nursing for many years without any problems like this and I felt my previous record was not taken properly into account.'

Because of this experience, Ms Farrell was particularly horrified when, eight months later, she realised she was responsible for a second mistake. A patient who had been prescribed a drug at 6 pm and 10 pm had the prescription reduced to 6 pm only while Ms Farrell was on her nights off duty. When she returned to the ward she 'automatically' gave the drug, again via a student nurse, at 10 pm.

She almost immediately realised a mistake had been made and rushed into the patient's side room to stop the student but was too late. Her feelings of frustration were increased because the student said the patient had queried the prescription. Ms Farrell feels the student should have then double checked.

She then made what she realises, in retrospect, was her biggest mistake. Because she had a written warning against her name, and was very concerned about the consequences of a second drug administration error within a year, she told the student not to mention the mistake. Four days later she did and Ms Farrell was called to account at a hospital hearing.

But this was only the beginning of her problems. Not only was she found guilty of the drug error, issued with a final written warning and forced to leave night duty, she was told that details of the case would be forwarded to the Investigating Committee of the English National Board. This Committee looks at the evidence and decides whether there is a case of professional misconduct to answer. If it believes there is, it forwards details to the UKCC Professional Conduct Committee.

In due course Ms Farrell learned that she would have to appear before the UKCC Committee and face the prospect of having her name removed from the Register of nurses and losing the right to practise as a nurse.

Her feelings at the time were understandably mixed. An awareness of the seriousness of the mistake she had made, and her folly in trying to cover it up, was mixed with anger towards the student who was involved, and ambivalent feelings about her employers.

'The student said a lot of nasty things about me,' she said. 'She accused me of roughing up a patient, of not being supportive and said that the patients did not like me.' Ms Farrell originally felt that the statements of complaint against her were so ludicrous as to be almost laughable but her RCN representative told her that things did not look particularly hopeful.

Ms Farrell believed her employers were anxious to discipline her but, paradoxically, appreciates they also seemed to care about her welfare. So much so that when, after the hospital inquiry, she wanted to resign, they would not accept the resignation.

'But I had to do a minimum of six months on day duty,' Ms Farrell said, 'and undertake a refresher course. I was not allowed to be in charge and could not be involved with giving drugs. The other staff were told both these things but were not told why.' Nevertheless, with the efficiency of most hospital grapevines, Ms Farrell has few doubts about the other staff knowing why these restrictions were made.

Towards the end of this six-month 'probationer' period, Ms Farrell had what she describes as a 'pseudopsychotic breakdown'.

She said, 'I was totally confused and in hospital for about five days. Even now that period is vague and only half remembered.' It is also a time Ms Farrell has difficulty talking about, because of the trauma involved in finding herself the recipient of psychiatric care.

From the time she was told that the details of her case would be forwarded to the ENB Investigating Committee until she appeared in front of the UKCC Professional Conduct Committee, about 11 months elapsed, which is quite quick as these things go. Initially, she was told the waiting time tends to be about two years.

When her case was eventually heard she was found guilty on two counts of administering the wrong drug (relating to the two separate incidents), of failing to report the errors and of discouraging a student from reporting the error. The Committee decided that, although professional misconduct was proved in all four incidents, no further action should be taken.

Ms Farrell said of the hearing, 'The Chairwoman was very nice and very fair. I felt the Committee was concerned about me and trying to get all the facts. My RCN representative was super but, throughout the whole thing, the people who helped most were the Nurses' Welfare Service.

'For me, the big problem is the medical history. I think that hospital admission is what will have the longest lasting effect. I am not surprised at what happened because I was so strung up and under such a strain that something had to give.'

The feeling of having an invaluable ally in the Nurses' Welfare Service is echoed by Frances Kelly, who also appeared before the UKCC Professional Conduct Committee. Unlike Ms Farrell, her misconduct did not relate to a practice-related offence but concerned a criminal offence, namely, defrauding a credit card company.

At a time of great emotional problems, Ms Kelly used a credit card fraudulently; probably in an effort to bolster her low spirits she admits. Having endured the embarrassment and shame of appearing in court – the outcome of which was a two year conditional discharge and order to repay the debts incurred – Ms Kelly received notification that she would be considered by the UKCC Professional Conduct Committee.

'This was rather a shock,' she said, 'as I had been unaware until then that the UKCC would be informed of my court appearance and subsequent conviction.' The sense of shock was exacerbated because Ms Kelly had got a job as a staff nurse but had not revealed her conviction, fearing it would jeopardise her chances. She needed to have a full time job to pay off the debts she had incurred fraudulently and to pay off other debts; bills which had caused her to use someone else's credit card in the first place.

'With assistance and invaluable advice from the Nurses' Welfare Service, I prepared a statement for the ENB Investigating Committee,' she said. The ENB decided there was a case to answer and details were forwarded to the UKCC. A few months later the UKCC forwarded a detailed list of the charges against Ms Kelly.

'During this period of waiting I was in contact with the NWS and had sessions with one of their counsellors,' she said. 'It was from this service that I learned most about the procedures I was about to be part of. They helped me prepare for my hearing and gave me much needed support.

'My professional misconduct case was heard about 13 months after I was told I was to be investigated. At the hearing a solicitor read out the charges against me and the members could then ask questions. In my case there was only one witness the UKCC had contacted to provide them with a character profile of my nursing ability and competency before the misconduct charges.

'I fully expected to be called to the witness stand and answer questions but, to my surprise, the Committee decided not to put me in the witness stand and the Chairman asked me only one question. They then retired to another room and, although the wait seemed to be a long time, it was only about 10 minutes. The

Chairman told me that, although found guilty of misconduct, my name would not be removed from the Register.

'The whole procedure had lasted about an hour and all I can remember directly afterwards is the tremendous feeling of relief and the great number of tears I cried.'

Ms Kelly, like Ms Farrell, felt the Committee was sympathetic and kind and tried to help her relax, as far as is possible under the circumstances.

'The only criticism I have is concerning the long delay between initially being informed I was being investigated and the case being heard. My case was heard quickly because the UKCC had asked if I was prepared to appear with less than 28 days' notice if another case was postponed. I agreed as I wanted the pressure to be gone, no matter what the outcome.

'The long period of waiting certainly affected me. I became very pessimistic and convinced that I would not be allowed to pursue my nursing career. This belief became so firm that, before the hearing took place, I gave up nursing.

'At the risk of sounding melodramatic I can honestly say there was not one day during this stressful and anxious waiting period that I did not have the hearing, and all it entailed, on my mind. This was particularly disturbing as I was also trying to come to terms with my feelings of shame and guilt at my criminal actions.'

Both Ms Kelly and Ms Farrell were struck with how similar to a courtroom is the room in which professional conduct cases are heard. They also agree on how exposed they felt. Another aspect of the hearing that disturbed them greatly was the fact that hearings are open to the public and are often attended by nurses who are there as observers.

One thing they did not experience was going to prison and having their names removed from the Register. But this happened to Margaret Clifton, whose story is told in the next section. Miss Clifton badly injured her back in a car accident and eventually became hooked on DF118 painkillers to the extent of stealing and forging prescriptions.

She said, 'After an article in *Nursing Times* I had a lot of letters from nurses with similar problems, particularly from men with alcohol-related problems. They all said they felt isolated and uncared for by the profession and as if they were the only ones with such a problem.

'I know that I could always ring the Nurses' Welfare Service, and often did, and they came to see me as often as possible, but it would have helped to have had someone on the spot.'

Because of her own experiences, Margaret has started a support group in Birmingham for nurses with drug or alcohol-related problems, believed to be the first such group of its kind in the country.

She is employed as a district drug abuse research worker, has spent much of her own time in recent years working for Drugline, a charity to help drug users, and believes her own experiences give her a unique perspective.

If you should ever receive a letter from your National Board saying the Investigating Committee is deciding whether there is a case of professional misconduct for you to answer, there are people you can turn to. It will not make the process easy, but it may make it easier.

Struck off. One nurse's story

by Harriet Gaze

Margaret Clifton was in prison serving a nine month sentence for theft and forgery when she was told by the Assistant Governor that she had been struck off the Register. She had not been allowed out of prison to attend her professional conduct hearing and was still suffering the after-effects of drug addiction.

In 1981, three years after her removal from the Register and the Midwives' Roll and following almost three years of unemployment, Miss Clifton was restored to the Register. She qualified as a health visitor, and Birmingham Central Health Authority wanted to create a specialist post for her working with drug abusers.

While Miss Clifton's remarkable story of a nurse who managed to turn her personal disaster into a success represents an extreme example of the difficulties which can face someone struck off the Register, the problems she faced were similar to those faced by anyone who has had their right to practise their profession removed.

Miss Clifton had been working as a midwifery sister before being struck off in 1978. She badly injured her back during a car crash on an American holiday, and when she returned to England still in pain, her GP prescribed DF118 (dihydrocodeine). Gradually she began to take the drug regardless of whether she was in pain or not, and this addiction led to theft and forgery of prescriptions. 'Basically, over a period of 15 months I became hooked on them. I knew all the time it would eventually lead to being struck off the Register but I just couldn't stop.'

By the time that Miss Clifton was finally sentenced to prison in October 1977 she had already been arrested several times and had been put on probation. Hearing that she had been struck off the Register while still trying to conquer her drug addiction was shattering. Sending her badge back to the General Nursing Council was also deeply upsetting.

'After 12 years of working as a nurse and my parents having been so proud of me when I qualified, it just devastated me, and I vowed I would get back, even if it took me 20 years.'

Losing the right to practise led to feelings of anger, shame and isolation. 'When you are struck of you feel you are the only person in the world in that position. You feel you are just in a bottomless pit and think, "Well, I am never going to get back".'

In particular she thought she had let down her parents, who had supported her throughout her various court appearances. 'I had caused them so much anguish and I just felt so ashamed of myself – I felt ashamed of everything.'

After her own experiences, Miss Clifton went about setting up a self help support group for nurses who have been struck off the Register in order to lessen the common sense of shame and isolation.

At the time of her removal from the Register, Miss Clifton also felt extremely bitter towards other nurses. 'Whenever I saw a nurse it was like a red rag to a bull. I eventually came to terms with it but it took me a long time. I just felt this deep resentment, and felt there were so many people who had committed offences and they had got off but I had got caught.'

These feelings were possibly partly caused by the psychological effects of coming off drugs, she thinks. But it also seems that they were the result of the lack of support she received from nursing colleagues during her addiction and from the nurses working in prison.

'When I was a midwifery sister and had started using drugs, they might have suspected it, but no one said anything.' She felt unable to bring the subject up with colleagues because of the consequences for her career. 'There is no way I could have gone up to a nurse and said "I am hooked on drugs".

35

'It is a sad reflection on nursing when people cannot admit they have a problem for fear of reprisal. Nurses are not a caring profession in that they don't care for each other.'

During the first months of her prison sentence she was cared for in the hospital wing while she withdrew from the drugs, but the attitude of the prison nurses was the opposite of supportive and she was described by some as 'a disgrace to the profession'.

Serving the sentence, however, first in Risley Remand Centre and then at Styal Prison, saved her life, according to Miss Clifton. Once out of the hospital wing she gained much friendship and support from the other prisoners.

Leaving prison and starting proper life again is much harder than serving the prison sentence, Miss Clifton claims. She was released in June 1978 – in time to attend the hearing at the Central Midwives Board and be struck off the Roll.

After an eight-week stint at a rehabilitation centre where a psychologist tried to persuade her that she would never nurse again, and over a year of unemployment, Miss Clifton became a founder member of Birmingham's Drugline – a counselling service for users, their friends and relations. She never did manage to find full time work but thinks that her Drugline experience encouraged the GNC to restore her to the Register in 1981.

The Nurses' Welfare Service provided a lifeline whenever she felt depressed, and helped her prepare for the traumatic restoration hearing.

Pent-up hope can make the restoral procedure as agonising as the original Professional Conduct Committee hearing. 'I went up for the hearing and I have never been so nervous in my life – I just felt sick.' And she did actually vomit before she arrived at the GNC headquarters.

In the event, Miss Clifton was restored to the Register. 'As I went out they handed me my badge and my certificate and I went out feeling I could have just shouted it to the world. I was elated for about two weeks, then the hard reality hit me – I still had to get a job.'

She visited a local nursing officer who was interested in helping nurses who had suffered drink or drug problems and he offered her nursing work in a geriatric hospital. 'He said, "I am giving you this job because I admire your honesty. It won't be common knowledge among your colleagues and if anybody knows it will be because you have told them".'

What colleagues would think of her if they knew her background was a major fear in the early days. On one later occasion when she was working as a midwife, she met a former colleague and was petrified that her past would be discovered. 'I went up to her and told her, and she said "I respect you now for telling me," and after that I was just treated like any other person.'

Miss Clifton has no qualms about what colleagues think of her past. 'I am not worried now about what people think because I have got back to work and I don't need to prove things with my colleagues – I did at first.'

Dealing with drugs also caused her some alarm: the attitudes of other nurses towards the checking process seemed appallingly lax. 'I wasn't prepared to let anything happen which would cause me to lose my registration again.'

Working with pethidine was particularly frightening for someone who had injected it in the course of her own drug addiction. Nurses were often reluctant to accompany her on drug rounds on the grounds that they 'trusted' her. She always made sure that she got a student nurse to come with her.

Miss Clifton went on to lecture to trainee health visitors at Birmingham Polytechnic on the problems of drug abuse. 'Whenever I give these talks, wherever I go to do a lecture, there is always somebody who comes up at the end – a nurse – who says they have had a problem with drink or drugs – tranquillisers most of the time.'

She also likes to talk to nurse learners about the professional conduct process and how easy it is to find oneself an unhappy participant in it.

Anyone who is struck off the Register is going to feel depressed and isolated, says Miss Clifton. 'But they must realise that people do get back on and there is hope. It is essential to make goals and to completely change your lifestyle if you are struck off.' She denies that she is a particularly strong person, but has realised how many hidden strengths she developed in order to survive.

Miss Clifton developed an enviable career in nursing based partly on her own original problems. 'I was quite impressed with the attitude of the people who employed me. When you are trying to get a job, be honest and go and see people first to talk to them because they will admire you for your honesty.'

The Committee member

Reviewing the evidence

by Isobel Morrison

As a member of the UKCC, I am often one of the five members of the Professional Conduct Committee (PCC). Most dates I know well ahead, but sometimes I am a reserve and keep a bag packed ready. The work contrasts greatly with what I do in Edinburgh as an enrolled nurse caring for elderly people.

About a week before a meeting of the PCC I receive the papers from the UKCC. These have a list of the cases – for each, the name of the respondent, date of birth, nursing qualification(s) with dates and places of training and the charges.

Reading these at home, and again the evening before the meeting, I note the age and likely experience of the nurse. Do I understand the charge? If the facts of the charge are not admitted, what do I need to know to be convinced of the facts? The wording of the charges, drawn up by Council's solicitors and officers, is very important. In coming to a decision as to whether or not there has been misconduct, we may concern ourselves only with what is contained in the charges.

Once the facts are proven, we have to decide if they constitute professional misconduct. Some do, for example, ill treatment of a patient. Others need more background for us to appreciate the full implications of the facts.

Professional Conduct Committee meetings are held in a formal setting complete with microphones. If I have butterflies in my stomach, how does a respondent feel? Sadly, some respondents are so overcome by the occasion they cannot do themselves justice. Members are sympathetic. They agree with the Irish nurse member who said, 'There, but for the grace of God, go I.'

As the case proceeds, witnesses give evidence, are questioned and cross-examined. Documents are submitted, statements are made. There are details of times, dates and places. Careful, constant concentration is needed. It rather frightened me at first that I knew I had to vote one way or another at three stages. First, are the facts proven? Second, is this professional misconduct? Third, what action is to be taken? No abstentions are allowed. It gave me early comfort to realise that the Chairman, before calling a vote in public or *in camera*, first asks if all members are ready to vote.

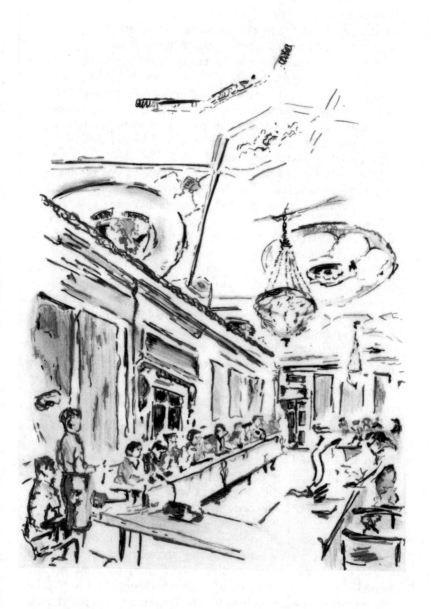

An artist's impression of a Professional Conduct Committee hearing in progress

The impossibility of abstention sharpens the mind. I find an early morning swim increases my span of attention. I write down verbatim some of the evidence, particularly the respondent's. I write down questions, ticking them off as the proceedings give answers. I underline and add asterisks.

Which evidence are we to believe? People notice events differently, concentrate on different aspects. Witnesses can disagree honestly. Can the inconsistencies be reconciled? Is a witness lying, prejudiced or unsure? One great difficulty is the amount of time that has since elapsed. Can witnesses remember the incident, or only what they have said before about it? Can they visualise what happened?

Witnesses have a hard time. They have to answer on oath questions from lawyers, union representatives and members of the Committee. Sad as it is to hear cases involving poor care or ill treatment of patients, there are encouraging factors, such as the reasons given for hesitation before the first reporting of an incident. Witnesses have been shocked and do not want to believe what they have seen – they have never seen anything like it before. Few like to speak against a colleague. All credit to those who do, putting the patient's interest first. All credit to those who are prepared to come and speak up for their colleagues.

What about the questions put by members of the Committee? At least one of us will have experience in the relevant field. My questions are likely to be on practical details drawing on my familiarity with bedside nursing. Sometimes I have a listening role only. The answers to other members' questions throw light on an unfamiliar field.

It is perhaps relatively easy to determine what is professional misconduct in a well staffed scene of excellent practice. Too often we are looking at areas where there are staff shortages, difficulty in obtaining equipment or supplies, and morale is low. Is something misconduct if it is general practice? Is the respondent a scapegoat? We need a full picture of the surrounding circumstances of the incident. If we stray too widely the legal assessor will be quick to limit our line of questioning.

When we are *in camera*, I do not necessarily have my mind made up. I may have questions and want to draw on the knowledge and experience of other members. There may be statements or references to read. The Chairman makes sure each member has a chance to speak and keeps debate to the issue in hand. Discussion may centre on advice given by the legal assessor, advice which is repeated in public. Different points of view emerge. As well as having particular expertise, we are members of the vulnerable public. Each case is unique, but the experience and recall of Council's officer helps to define the pertinent issues. We try to build up a full picture of the incident and of the respondent.

Where it becomes obvious there are opposing views, I try to understand why a particular view is held. I try to make clear the reasons for my opinion. After full discussion, which may explain why we are sometimes a long while *in camera*, I am content to accept a majority vote. A unanimous decision is perhaps the most common.

The standards against which to assess professional conduct are those it is reasonable to expect, not the best. Some cases have charges concerned with events outside work. A nurse completely out of control of her private life is unlikely to be in safe control of her working life. There are less extreme cases. The Committee's concern is for the special relationship the nurse has with the vulnerable public. People cannot usually choose who will nurse them. It is the UKCC's job not only to establish standards of education for a nurse, but also to be satisfied she is a fit person to nurse. 'Of good character' is the phrase used in the 1979 Act (Section 11, clause (2)). That is why 'conduct unworthy of a nurse', difficult as this is to assess, is misconduct.

It is at the stage of mitigation/aggravation (reached after misconduct is proven) that we look perhaps most closely at the respondent. What is the respondent's nursing record? Everybody can produce mitigating evidence; we all have problems. But was help available, offered and refused? Was help sought but not forthcoming? Under stress the nurse did something wrong, or omitted to do something that should have been done. We are assured it will never happen again. Has the respondent worked out a way of coping with future stress? Has anything changed? Has the respondent learned from the experience? Has she gained insight? What has the respondent been doing meanwhile? Has she been nursing successfully? The business of the Committee is to protect the vulnerable public, not to punish. Indeed, Society may have already exacted the punishment of imprisonment.

I have come to value the work of the Nurses' Welfare Service. At first, knowing the respondent has the right of representation, I saw the service as an unnecessary extra. It is not that the

41

welfare officers give the respondents the right answers. They, and some probation officers, seem able to help a nurse look at themselves, accept what has happened and start rebuilding – walking before running.

The respondent is sometimes a loner. The loner has an initial realisation of something being wrong. Events get out of control because of a failure to talk through the difficulty; perhaps because they are away from home, working in an unfamiliar setting, not understanding a new culture.

Management and colleagues may have tried unsuccessfully to bridge the gap. It is sometimes only removal from the Register that makes a person realise there are problems to be tackled. How rewarding it is for members of the PCC (and a welfare officer if involved) when an applicant comes to the Committee and shows she is fit to be restored to the Register and will no longer put the public at risk.

During the course of hearing evidence, it may emerge that much is wrong with the situation over and above the charges in front of us. It can be very frustrating to have to listen to descriptions of undesirable practice. The UKCC sends transcripts of proceedings which reveal poor conditions, staff shortages and bad practice to the relevant Health Authorities.

What conclusions do I draw from PCC work? The composition of the Committee achieves a balance of experience and opinion. Observers see that the whole nursing situation is looked at and that respondents are treated kindly and given every chance. Even though respondents have usually been through inquiries and/or court proceedings, new evidence emerges.

Procedure has improved with experience gained since 1983, and will further improve as rule changes are achieved. This success is in large part due to the skill and dedication of Council's officer and staff.

The length of time elapsing after an incident before being heard by the PCC is not acceptable; it should be a year at most. It is inevitable that some decisions of the Committee will be wrong. However, the PCC is doing, and is seen to be doing, a reasonable and fair job.

I hope that the presence of an enrolled nurse member, with current 'hands on' experience, encourages respondents and witnesses. As an enrolled nurse I may have a bias against management. Even so, my comments on some managers may be valid. I am concerned at attitudes to mistakes, a lack of sympathy. Is there a nurse who has not made a mistake? What matters most is that the mistake is admitted quickly, reported to the person who has the knowledge and experience to assess its importance and is able to implement speedily any necessary remedial action. Do managers wish to encourage admission of mistakes? Worry about over-reaction to minor mistakes may be the cause of 'cover-ups' and major mistakes. Dealing with a self-reported mistake is surely a matter of management and not of professional conduct.

I would like to mention one particular case. A charge nurse trained over 20 years ago had mentally ill patients in his care. His nurse manager was concerned that the charge nurse was not adopting modern methods of care. Many attempts to help him had failed. A newly trained enrolled nurse was put on the charge nurse's shift in the hope of proving a good influence. The EN later gave evidence in court of the ill treatment of a patient by that charge nurse. The EN has since left that hospital. I do not know why but I am not surprised.

My experience on the PCC has convinced me that there will always be, unnecessary as it is, such misuse of enrolled nurses. Because of this, I endorse Project 2000's proposal to stop training *more* enrolled nurses. I see clearly, as ever, a useful role for present enrolled nurses.

Looking at the UKCC's final Project 2000 proposals I have high hopes that attitudes will change, that as a result nurses will be better managers, better managed, and more appropriately deployed. The vulnerable public will be less at risk and will benefit.

Colleagues

Blowing the whistle

by Derek McCarthy

It is likely that at sometime during your career you could be accused of an abuse against a patient or, at least, will witness such an event perpetrated by a colleague. It may be that you have already witnessed an abuse and that this has troubled your conscience.

If you have – and if other nurses' experiences are anything to go by – you will have had considerable difficulties in coping with the situation. In the end you may have done the right thing and reported the matter officially, but in that case you would be in a minority. Most of us tend to be overcome by the difficulties and pressures associated with making complaints against colleagues and keep quiet.

These pressures were first identified by Virginia Beardshaw in *Conscientious Objectors at Work*[1]. Conscientious objectors are usually associated with those who choose for religious or ethical reasons not to fight in wars, but she applies the term to staff who object to certain practices which infringe individual rights. She includes a checklist of 24 points for 'whistle blowers', a colloquialism for those who contemplate making such a complaint.

The issues raised by Virginia Beardshaw's work were the subject of a NAHA working party under Julia Cumberlege, then Chairman of Brighton Health Authority (Virginia Beardshaw acted as its project officer).

That report[2] was published in 1985 and made recommendations which apply to all specialties, but with emphasis on long-stay, high-dependency patients. This is sensible: abuse of patients, at one time endemic in the mental illness/mental handicap field, has reduced significantly, and now seems to be fairly equally distributed through all specialties. There are, however, strong indications that staff in general hospitals have greater difficulties than their colleagues in mental illness/mental

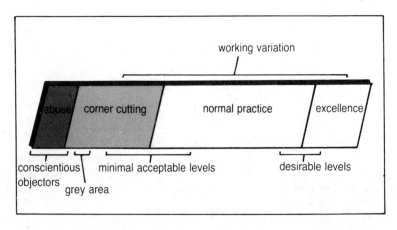

Spectrum of care

handicap services in discussing abuse openly or bringing it to the attention of their managers.

This is partly because nurses find it hard to place the nature of abuse into perspective. There is a tendency to meander into the entire spectrum of care, of standard setting, quality control and monitoring. All of these are important and relevant to abuse, but they are too large and complex to look at collectively. There is a tendency to produce documents which say something about everything but very little that is of practical help to frontline staff.

The above figure illustrates the full spectrum of care; the normal working variations which take into account differing levels of workload and fluctuations in manpower/skill levels. On the far left is the narrow area of abuse which is the concern of 'conscientious objectors'.

There are five main categories of abuse.

1. Physical abuse: from rough handling to punching, slapping and kicking, or worse.
2. Sexual abuse: forcing or promoting unwelcome sexual attention or practices.
3. Psychological abuse: causing emotional distress by verbal means, such as badgering, demeaning, coercing, provoking or frightening, or by making someone undertake or witness acts which are personally distasteful.
4. Neglect/deprivation: deliberately withholding basic rights and comforts such as food, light, heat, personal hygiene and contact with others.
5. Misappropriation of personal effects: stealing money, valuables, articles with sentimental attachments or any other personal belongings.

There is also a grey area (shown in the figure) between abuse and corner cutting, where it is much more difficult to agree on guilt. 'Corner cutting' is a euphemism often used by nurses and others to describe a universal and time honoured practice, where work is undertaken at a faster pace and at a lower standard than normal, usually in times of crisis. As a result some patients receive less attention, either for the ultimate benefit of those who require more, or for the total benefit of the group as a whole.

Allegations against staff which fall into this grey area require knowledgeable, searching and sensitive investigations, since the ultimate fault may not lie with the individual but may be, in whole or in part, the result of poor management.

The figure opposite takes the area of abuse shown in the previous figure and gives some indication of the nature and extent of the problem; what is known (both officially and unofficially) and what is unknown – undoubtedly the largest and most difficult part of the problem to deal with.

What then are the difficulties associated with making complaints? A lack of clear written guidance to staff on how to make a complaint is usually seen as the major problem. Therefore, in theory, once clear policy guidelines are introduced, the situation should improve.

However it is often those with least knowledge of organisational structures and policies who actually 'blow the whistle' – that is, new members of staff, students, nursing assistants and domestics. Frequently senior staff, who know precisely what they should do, remain silent or try to obstruct those who are intending to complain.

But other difficulties inhibit complaints and these need to be more fully understood. Only by carefully discussing these issues with staff will nurse managers be able to diminish the levels of abuse. Nurses need to know about the enormous personal, group and social pressures when they are contemplating making a complaint.

Few staff make unfounded or malicious complaints against colleagues. A predictable response from the accused is that the allegations are motivated out of jealousy, to repay a personal grudge or are just the product of a personality conflict. Where more than one person is making allegations, collusion with the same motivation is often suggested. In reality, this is rare – few staff would embark on the difficult and tortuous course of making serious fictitious complaints against colleagues knowing they too will come under the scrutiny of an internal hospital inquiry, police investigation, National Board disciplinary inquiry or a Health Authority Appeals Committee, or a combination of these.

Staff making complaints usually act out of a genuine abhorrence of bad practice and in an attempt to protect those in their care, knowing that otherwise the bad practice could well continue.

It is generally easier to complain where there is a tradition of open management, where there is a culture which supports

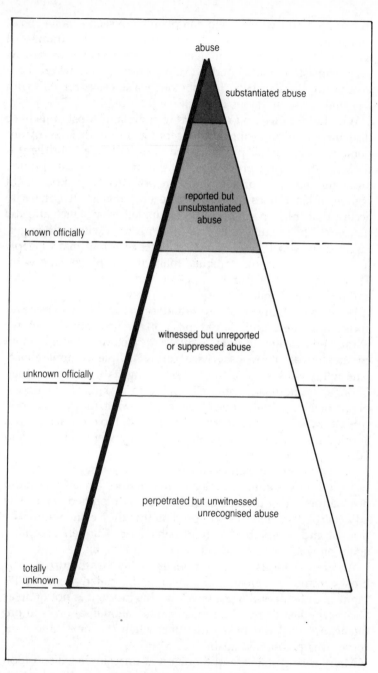

Extent of the problem of abuse

free speech and where valid complaints are seen as a means of improving practice. It is also helpful when the traditional working divide between 'managers' and 'workers' is as narrow as is consistent with good working practice and where both groups are close socially. It is obviously also easier for staff with a strong sense of values and self confidence.

Why then do we find it so hard to complain? Most of us have difficulty in recognising and accepting the 'dark side' of our personalities. We all prefer to see ourselves in a good light – those in the caring profession believe in their special aptitude and motivation to protect and care for the sick, although of course, most nurses agree they are not 'angels'. It is hard to accept that 'nice' people can be fascinated by violence and the macabre. The mixture of feelings – revulsion, excitement, anger, fascination, shock, sorrow and impotence – that many people feel when witnessing an abuse make it difficult to cope with. They expect to be purely repelled and are not prepared for ambivalent feelings.

When asked, most of us would say that we would never abuse a patient and would promptly report any abuse we witnessed. Reality paints a different picture. Under certain circumstances many otherwise caring people commit abuse. And many abuses are witnessed by caring staff, some over long periods, without anyone feeling able to make a 'formal complaint' or even to make their objections known to the perpetrators.

Staff who have witnessed abuses and took no action will admit to a variety of ways in which they were able to avoid taking appropriate action.

Denial is one response and in some cases is absolute. The nurse witnesses abuse but is able to convince herself that it did not happen. In other cases the denial is modified. Here she adjusts the facts in her own mind so that they come within the normal and acceptable range of behaviour. This self deception again allows her to avoid action or confrontation.

Another response is to rationalise what has occurred. The most common rationalisations include 'the patient deserved it', 'he was difficult and aggressive' or 'this incident is not quite as bad as the last I saw'. The most classic rationalisation is to put off action until the next time, and when the next time does come, it is postponed again.

Many caring staff are of a quiet and unassuming disposition and lack self confidence. Accordingly they may find it extremely difficult to report a working colleague, particularly if that person is an 'authority figure'. Sometimes women are reluctant to report their male colleagues.

Whatever the initial reason, once a person has witnessed an incident and has not reported it, it becomes progressively more difficult for them to do so when it happens again. They start to believe they have colluded in some way with bad practice and fear that, should the situation become public, it will reflect adversely on them.

In well established teams most people are on good terms. The abuser may be a friend or a good working colleague – making an allegation will break the friendship and may tarnish their reputation or lose them their livelihood.

Some nurses may be reluctant to approach their managers if they doubt whether impartial and vigorous action would be taken. Junior staff may also believe that their lack of status and experience will lead to managers automatically 'taking the word' of someone senior. If the managers have never discussed these matters frankly and openly with their staff, then these feelings will persist. There are, alas, some managers who feel that anything wrong within their sphere of responsibility reflects badly on them and are more interested in promoting a good image than opening up issues of bad practice.

Nurses also witness abuses by doctors and many experience greater difficulty in reporting them. Doctors are assumed to have superior status, intellectual capacity and knowledge. Their position is also virtually unassailable. Their rules allow for much greater latitude in personal behaviour and practice. Moreover the application of these rules takes an extraordinary time to achieve results compared with those for other workers.

Almost everyone who reports colleagues for ill treatment is a member of a staff organisation, a fact which officials of these organisations sometimes find it inconvenient to acknowledge. It makes their lives more difficult if they have to support both accused and the accuser.

It is simpler to stand only behind the accused and to play out the old charade of managers against workers. The inquiry then becomes a straightforward 'them' and 'us' conflict, making the establishment of the facts more difficult.

It would be more helpful if both managers and unions could accept that each has equal responsibility for protecting and supporting all patients and staff, upholding good standards and improving services.

For anyone contemplating a complaint against a colleague, it must be the ultimate irony to know that their own staff organisation may not give full support and could even be instrumental in casting doubt on their reliability and competence. All staff involved should be made aware of their rights to be represented, supported and protected by their staff organisation. Although this might complicate the situation for staff organisations and managers, it would help to remove the well founded fears among many that their professional body automatically sides with the accused.

In any hospital we should know the number and nature of reported abuses which are acted on by senior managers and the result of their interventions. But what of the witnessed events which go unreported or are suppressed? In these cases knowledge is very limited. From my own experience many nurses (with often only a few years service) have witnessed acts of abuse which concerned them and yet they felt unable to take appropriate action in accordance with their consciences. And of course we know absolutely nothing about acts perpetrated in the absence of witnesses or where the abused patient is unable or unwilling to report the matter, and for which there is no other detectable evidence available.

If we consider the pyramid in the previous figure again, it is not unreasonable to postulate that the total level of abuse is likely to be greater than we have realised. So for the future protection of patients, the following recommendations should be made to health authorities and managers.

- All authorities should include in their staff handbook a clear statement on conscientious objectors at work which includes comprehensive guidelines for staff who witness abuse.
- A number of staff should be selected from management, personnel and education, to train other senior managers on a district-wide basis.
- Once trained, managers should organise multidisciplinary training sessions on a continuous basis for all staff.

References

1 Beardshaw, V. *Conscientious Objectors at Work*. London: Social Audit, 1981.
2 NAHA. *Protecting Patients*. Birmingham: NAHA, 1985.

4

The Problems

An accident waiting to happen

All too often nurses are expected to make supreme efforts to cope with poor conditions related to the environment of care. However, it is not wise to struggle on, in silence, bearing the burden of understaffing, overcrowding and taking short cuts with hazardous practices. Such a level of functioning leaves both staff and patients vulnerable, by making the nurse's workload personally intolerable and professionally dangerous.

" Saturday night and the relief staff midwife had rung in sick – again. I was told a replacement would be sent but was not surprised when no one appeared. We were left to muddle on as usual, five of us struggling to do the work of six, with more babies than the unit had been designed for.

As the senior midwife, sister on the special care baby unit (SCBU), I was the only permanent full time member of staff on night duty. Part time staff midwives Lake and Singh were familiar with the unit but were allocated where they were most needed in the department. That night I also had a new agency midwife and an enrolled nurse, borrowed from the antenatal ward.

The unit had filled up since my last spell of nights, with cots and accompanying equipment crammed closely together; it was difficult to move around. Of course, we understand the dilemma; if babies aren't accepted, they have no chance of survival. We are their only hope but it doesn't make our job any easier. With 17 babies crowded into space meant for 13, the overstretching of staff and facilities was near to danger point.

Several mothers were good at helping out by giving the last evening feed, but they needed to get their rest.

Individualised patient care was something of a joke here at night. Patient allocation could work, up to a point, but it took only one slow feeder or other problem to throw good plans awry. Because

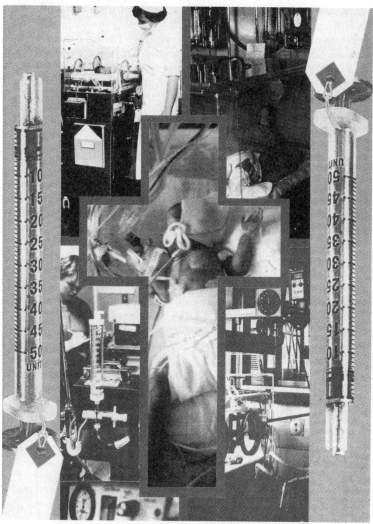

the staff were thinly spread anyone had to be able to respond to any baby and tasks fell to whoever was available.

The clock dictated nurses' movements as they worked, repetitiously attending to the needs of many babies; observation, nappy, handwash, feed, turn, handwash and so on. I found it much easier to delegate one nurse as the runner, dealing with support tasks collectively. Two midwives were allocated to the ventilated babies and those with critical observations, infusions and monitors. Another nurse worked in the cot bay round the corner on nursery duties, helped by the other when available. With our good teamwork, we pulled together in this medley of unrelenting tasks in critical care nursing.

When mealtimes came, the cycle was speeded up between fewer nurses. Sometimes we had help from down the corridor but not that night. Nurses were often willing to miss their meal time but I always insisted they leave the unit. Mind you, I rarely managed more than a snatched cup of coffee in the parents' lounge.

Although it is always high dependency work, on that Saturday we were especially busy. There were two tots on ventilators, six babies in incubators, one under phototherapy, together with five intravenous infusions and several nasogastric tubes needing attention.

Baby Sims had been with us for a month. Originally weighing in at just over 1kg, he was making good progress and, although now off the ventilator, was being nursed in an incubator. He had a scalp vein infusion, nasogastric feeding, cardiac monitoring and constant oxygenation because he was still prone to attacks of apnoea.

By 11 pm staff midwife Lake was up to date with her work and it seemed an ideal opportunity to send her for a meal break. She had prepared the next round of tube feeds and put the syringes on each relevant incubator. All the nurses were so familiar with this routine that it seemed unnecessary to label the containers individually.

After S/M Lake had gone news came that a baby would be due soon following an emergency Caesarian section, so I was busily preparing to receive him.

Meanwhile, S/M Singh, who was attending baby Sims' routine care, noticed tissuing of his intravenous infusion. This line was carrying both parentrovite and intralipid.

I quickly got together another intravenous line. Baby Sims was running out of suitable sites and the doctor didn't think the lumen of the new blood vessel would be able to acommodate a multiple fluid input.

The white intralipid had been given from a syringe mounted in a pump, which was on top of the incubator. Beside the pump lay the low birth weight solution in readiness for nasogastric feeding – also a white fluid in a syringe.

The doctor stopped the intralipid and sealed the inlet to the Y-intravenous line. He wrote a new infusion regime which meant the two fluids would be alternated.

Our new baby was collected from the labour suite and admitted by S/M Lake, who had relieved S/M Singh. I took over baby Sims' observations and checked that the new drip site was working well. As the parentrovite was nearly through and the intralipid was due I attached the charged syringe to the infusion.

Assured that the staff were coping, I grabbed some tea and toast in the office while dealing with the new admission paperwork.

I was interrupted by the agency midwife, concerned that baby Sims was having breathing difficulties. I instituted half-hourly observations. The other midwives made the subsequent two checks and neither suspected any obvious complication. When the apnoeic attacks became increasingly frequent and persistent, I called the doctor, who was equally bewildered.

Nobody could understand the sudden distress and deterioration in this baby's condition. Our repeated attempts at resuscitation failed. Without a known cause we were working blind. Baby Sims died without explanation.

Not until the post mortem was it discovered that the low birth weight feed syringe had been attached to the intravenous line with subsequent tragic consequences.

The awful reality of my action was devastating. I was stunned by disbelief, followed by overwhelming sorrow and regret.

I had to admit to this unfortunate error but argued that my mistake, under extreme duress, did not **99** amount to professional misconduct.

Think points

- What part of the Code is under question here?
- What factors contributed to this tragic event?
- Identify the safety hazards in this unit.
- Discuss measures that could be recommended to improve safety and the delivery of patient care on this unit.
- What procedure should a nurse follow in refusing to accept more patients than she can safely care for?
- Using your judgement, do you consider that the sister could be accused of professional misconduct?

The official decision, and discussion

Part 11 of the Code of Professional Conduct states that, 'Each registered nurse, midwife and health visitor, in the exercise of professional accountability, shall have regard to the workload of and the pressures on professional colleagues and subordinates and take appropriate action if these are seen to be such as to constitute abuse of the individual practitioner and/or to jeopardise safe standards of practice.'

Detailed information about the operation of this unit revealed circumstances that amounted to dangerous practice. Gross overcrowding and critical understaffing presented severe nursing problems. There were few permanent care staff, midwives were allocated as needs demanded and allowed. On the night in question the unit had been meant to have one more midwife but she was sent to the busy labour ward. It was normal practice, known to the senior manager, that charged syringes were not labelled.

Evidence was heard from expert witnesses about the management of such units. They reported that, even in a unit which was well designed, 18 babies of this degree of dependence would require a staff of not less than seven. Those staff would need to be deployed to maintain continuity of observation and care, which would necessitate the allocation of several babies to each trained member of staff. When they were shown photographs of the unit, the witnesses said it was grossly overcrowded in a way which would render good care and observation difficult, require more staff to achieve it, and make patient allocation even more important.

The Committee was gravely concerned by the appalling circumstances and the blatantly obvious hazards to patients and staff existing in this unit, particularly as the managers were aware of dangerous practices. After very long discussion it did not regard the sister as guilty of misconduct and the case was closed. In their opinion the midwife was as much a victim as the deceased baby. She was working in a place where an accident was waiting to happen.

Double fault

To err may be human but attempting to conceal a mistake is foolhardy. And, in the responsible capacity of a professional nurse, such a misguided, reckless act could spell potential disaster. Of course, there is enormous temptation to try to cover up a mistake and avoid detection, coupled with the anxiety, confusion and sheer disbelief of the moment. Some people may have other compelling reasons, such as superior personal standards that cannot concede to human failing, fear of a job in jeopardy, loss of face, dread of shame and notoriety. When pride and vanity get in the way of acceptable professional behaviour, the principle holds good, to 'own up, don't cover up'.

66 At the best of times, the theatre suite at Queen Anne's Hospital was notoriously busy. It needed a tight and effective routine, with cohesive teamwork, to keep pace with the steady flow of work.

We were also responsible for supervising student nurses and theatre course members. As a respected senior sister, I was keen to ensure that they received first-class training when assigned to my area. Many viewed me as a strict task master, because I tested them on individual instruments and operation sets, but I took pride in influencing their correct grasp of theatre techniques. After all, you cannot be too careful in our type of work, I am forever repeating.

I frequently overheard remarks about my 'obsessional' attention to detail, but these hurtful remarks were vindicated by the approval of surgeons who appreciated my exactness.

Mr Lawson for example, who could become most irate when delegated inept staff, had particularly requested that I be available to scrub for him. In confidence, he stated that he found me competent to manage his long and varied lists.

Other nurses seemed annoyed, maybe even jealous, that Mr Lawson had singled me out. Nevertheless, I had worked extensively in theatres in major hospitals, at home and abroad, and was, undeniably, the most experienced sister on the floor.

On Wednesdays, Theatre 3 was known jokingly as 'The Conveyor Belt', as two hectic general lists working back-to-back, crammed in as many patients as they could. The surgeons were seemingly unconcerned that the rapid turnover stretched the resources of the recovery ward and our theatre, both functioning well beyond the time when the bulk of staff had gone off duty.

When I arrived on the late shift there was already evidence of the preceding busy morning, with debris from the first list piled in the sluice room. I wasn't feeling one hundred per cent after a late night and some rather disturbed sleep. I yawned, stretched and changed in readiness for the next session.

Mr Lawson would be arriving promptly at 1pm, scrubbed, gowned and hollering for his greens to be tied. We hurriedly prepared the theatre, as patient number one was already in the anaesthetic room. This cholecystectomy was the first of many operations from the list which stretched interminably ahead of us.

As the hours ticked away, the patients came and went; cut, cured and repaired, as the surgeons deftly healed each presenting problem. Meanwhile, the back-up nursing team lent its vital support, supplying the necessary items in the specific order each was called for; 'drape', 'towels', 'clips', 'scalpel', 'forceps' . . . And I was there, anticipating every request.

Junior staff assisted with the many nonsterile run-around duties; taking path. specimens, collecting infusion bags, marking blood loss and hanging up used swabs. Following our normal theatre regime, I double-checked swabs with the swab nurse before she disposed of them, but the responsibility for instrument check rested with me alone.

As usual, Mr Lawson took the briefest of midway breaks, sufficient for a cup of tea, a call of nature and a hasty cigarette for the needy. The indomitable surgeon was soon urging us to carry on.

My legs ached fearfully from the continuous standing, my head was itching from the cap and, although the face mask was uncomfortable, it usefully shielded my occasional yawns.

At last, the end was in sight. What a relief; only one more patient to go. Just as Mr Lawson got underway on the final case, his senior registrar called from A&E. 'Acute abdomen, elderly gent in a bad way. Can we fit him in, Sister?'

No problem. Here was a seriously ill man of advancing years, whose life was undoubtedly saved by emergency intervention to relieve the offending obstruction.

Eventually the day was over and I smartly cleared the linen and put my last set of instruments into the automatic washer. At handover I informed the night staff nurse that the abdomen set would subsequently be ready for repacking. I checked my watch. Ten o'clock already. By the time I'd travelled home, there would just be time for a bath and a decent night's sleep before a new day began. It was always such a rush, an early duty following on after a late shift.

Back in theatre the following day, I was greeted by the night nurse with some fanciful tale. She and her colleague, so she said, on checking the instruments of the abdomen set, had found it short of one pair of Dunhill forceps. Not knowing whether she would be seeing me that morning, she had written a large, bold note and fixed it to the incomplete set. However, as she was able to report her findings to me personally, she left the matter for me to deal with.

Impossible! A full set of instruments went into the washer, I assured her. *She* must have made some mistake, because I was always meticulous when checking equipment. In 10 years of unblemished service to theatre nursing, never had a doubt been cast over my reputation.

Of course, I know full well what it's like for those girls on night shift, probably snatching sleep in the day, coming to work dog tired and hoping for a quiet night. They hurry to clear the work, ferociously checking instruments, counting swabs, folding linen like machines, while they chat earnestly about domestic trivia and boyfriends. It wouldn't be difficult for something to slip past their notice while they are gossiping. And it is not unknown for instruments to be inadvertently sent to the laundry or discarded into the rubbish sacks.

Anyway, it was inconceivable that I could have made such a simple mistake, not a chance. Check, check and check again has always been my motto, as well the students know.

After the nurses had gone off duty, I screwed up their notice and put it in my pocket. I had to make good the deficient set of instruments but decided not to bother contacting the nursing officer. Adhering strictly to the regulations, I was supposed to check with my senior manager if it were necessary to draw a replacement instrument from the reserve stock cupboard. But another busy day lay ahead with the gynaecological list; I did not want to make a fuss, so I helped myself to a spare pair of forceps to complete the abdomen set.

The night nurses made no further mention of the incident and I dismissed it as a minor confusion, not worthy of involving other members of staff. Then, two weeks later, I heard that the elderly gentleman successfully operated on for an acute obstruction had been making excellent progress, when he died unexpectedly. The post mortem confirmed the cause was a pulmonary embolism. During the autopsy, however, the pathologist also found a pair of Dunhill forceps lodged in the patient's abdomen.

When the matter was investigated, all the records were correct. As the inquiry deepened, the night nurses described the incident of the missing instrument. I admitted to replacing a pair of forceps from the reserve stock without the required check and explained why.

The health authority took a serious view of my action, dismissed me from my post immediately, and referred the matter to the ENB. They alleged that I had behaved irresponsibly when the instrument was reported missing and acted inappropriately to conceal the incident.

My representative and I argued that the fault lay with the hospital standard practice, where the responsibility for the instrument check rests solely with the instrument nurse in charge of that operation.

I found it unbelievable that my credibility and integrity as a nurse could be brought into disrepute. Never before had my managers cause to question my work. To my credit, I had 10 years impeccable, flawless service.

Aggrieved by my sudden loss of employment and income, and knowing I would have a long wait to be called before a Professional Conduct Committee hearing, I searched elsewhere for a job. A private hospital was delighted to welcome me to their staff. A fully trained, highly experienced theatre nurse with impressive curriculum vitae and glowing open references – they didn't waste time going through the formality of chasing a reference from my previous employer.

I saw no reason to give details of my dismissal or the ugly incident which threatened to blight my career. I felt certain that the allegations would not be substantiated, and that my **99** professional reputation would be cleared.

Think points

- Which part of the Code is under question in this case?
- Could you suggest safeguards in this department which might have prevented this regrettable incident?
- Identify factors which could contribute to or account for a nurse making a mistake in the execution of her professional duties.
- In your place of work, what course of action should you take if you were to make a mistake?
- Discuss the reasons which may tempt nurses to cover up mistakes in their professional practice.
- What lessons are there for nurse managers from this story?
- Using your judgement, do you consider that this sister could be accused of misconduct?

The official decision, and discussion

After careful consideration, the Committee decided to postpone judgement for three months (the shortest possible period of postponement), and asked that, for the resumed hearing, a reference be supplied from the respondent's new employer which had to be written with knowledge of the facts.

Part 2 of the Code of Professional Conduct states that, 'Each registered nurse, midwife and health visitor, in the exercise of professional accountability, shall ensure that no action or omission on his/her part or within his/her sphere of influence is detrimental to the condition or safety of patients/clients.'

This Committee would almost certainly have forgiven a genuine mistake made under pressure at the end of a busy day. But it could not forgive dishonesty of actions when the missing instrument was brought to the respondent's notice.

It seemed to be a case in which pride came before the patient's best interest.

By the time of the hearing, the respondent had a post as a theatre sister, seemingly obtained without references being taken up.

Although she presented the Committee with an excellent open reference concerning her competence as a theatre nurse from her new employer, it became clear during questioning that the reference had been written without knowledge of the incident which led the respondent to this hearing.

The Committee added that the response of the two night nurses had been less than adequate, although it was probably fairly typical of what might be expected from the average registered nurse.

One favourable outcome resulted from this hearing, for the hospital policy now stipulates an instrument check by two nurses in theatres.

A web of deceit and lies

It is absolutely crucial to the nursing profession that patients can feel entirely secure and confident with the practitioners allocated to deliver their care. In a role that naturally involves personal, close and confidential interaction, nurses must behave in a way that fosters trust. It is all too easy to spot opportunities where an unscrupulous nurse might abuse her confidential position and turn privileged information to her personal advantage, while disregarding the patient's rights.

66 We like to think of Fernleigh as a home from home for confused elderly clients who not only struggle with memory loss and emotional difficulties, but are mostly lonely and unsupported.

For many of these old people our day centre offers a lifeline of help, interest and companionship, and the chance of a hot square meal. Apart from their visits to us, they may see no one else and are often too disorganised or disoriented to remember to prepare food.

These frail old folk are treated atrociously by their relatives, who keep a clear distance and skirt around their responsibilities – until the time comes to benefit from a will! In essence, we become their new family and aim to provide a warm welcome into a caring environment. It's first name terms here, and the kettle is constantly on the boil.

I love my job as deputy sister and find it one of the more rewarding roles since completing my training in mental nursing. Phyllis, the social worker, and Tom, the charge nurse, share the supervision of the centre. I'm only too happy to leave the management side and paperwork to them because I've always preferred working directly with the clients.

I'm there to receive the old folk as they arrive each morning. You will find me organising mealtimes to ensure they get adequate nourishment; many of those with poor concentration or an added physical infirmity need help with eating and drinking.

I spearheaded fundraising to equip a laundry room to help with their washing and arranged a store of spare clothing to provide for the needy. We try to stir their memories, raise their spirits, get them oriented to reality and encourage integration through social activities.

We are not confined to the centre, and follow up patients in their own home if they are ill or confused and unable to join us. I like to volunteer for home visits, as I've built up a good rapport with our clients. Undoubtedly, our individualised service extends beyond the normal boundaries of simple day care.

The key to our successful, happy community lies in effective management and good teamwork, which includes a part time

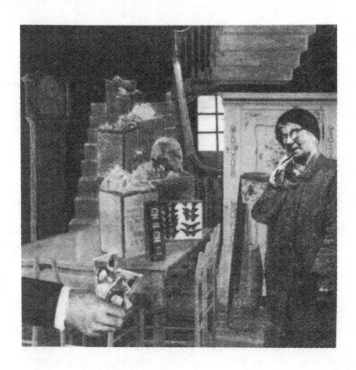

occupational therapist, and an enthusiastic bunch of community workers. These are mostly young people embarking on their first jobs, so I take them under my wing and train them in the correct ways. My concern is to maintain the quality of hands-on care.

Take Mark, for example, fresh up from the West Country in search of a job in London. He has proved immensely popular. He is an exceptional young man, who has shown a natural flare, with enduring patience and understanding for clients who are often difficult and cantankerous. For one so young, he has demonstrated a refreshingly keen attitude, interest and empathy in his new role.

Lily Day took a liking to him straightaway and, as one of our longstanding clients, put in a rightful claim to monopolise the 'new boy'. They would pass many a happy hour on recollections of pre-war England and the days of burlesque. The friendship helped the old lady through grief when her best friend died.

Winter brought new problems for Lily. Eighty years of age, frail and unsteady on her feet, it was a liability to leave her alone in her huge Victorian house, which was far too large for her simple needs. It was damp and draughty, yet, like many old people anxious about running up heating bills, Lily survived with a one-bar electric fire in her sitting-room-cum-bedroom. Because she was isolated in rambling overgrown grounds, Lily rightly feared burglary and attack, so would lock herself in, day and night.

It was not altogether surprising when Lily succumbed to hypothermia and had to be admitted to hospital. Although she made a good recovery, her mental state had deteriorated. Following assessment that also considered social circumstances, it was proposed that she be offered supervised accommodation. Naturally, Lily was reluctant to leave the home she had loved for 50 years. However, once she'd been to the site, she could appreciate the advantages of a compact, clean and cosy flatlet with modern conveniences and a caring warden.

Because Lily was incapable of handling her affairs, all her business was conducted through a solicitor, who was an agent of the Court of Protection. There was much activity involved with the move, too much for a confused old lady to manage. It involved the sale of the house with an estate agent and prospective buyers calling, settlement of outstanding bills and the disposal of many excess possessions.

We were keen to minimise the disturbance and to support Lily over this hurdle, knowing how change and upheaval can exacerbate confusion in the elderly. One colossal task was to sort and clear the belongings she had amassed over a lifetime. The team assigned myself, assisted by Mark, to make several visits to help Lily decide which furniture and personal trinkets would be appropriate for her new home.

The expanse of goods she owned had to be seen to be believed; masses of furniture, old clothes and linen, cooking utensils and a garden shed bursting with ancient tools. Admittedly much of the stuff was junk that could be dumped, but there were plenty of useful items that could be sold. Some pieces of furniture were beautifully crafted, with fine veneers.

The spare furniture was to be sold at auction, arranged by the solicitor, who would handle the proceeds of the sale on Lily's behalf. Lily was understandably distressed to see much of her past simply abandoned. She found it hard to make a definite choice especially of the framed pictures, and became tearful and nostalgic as we stacked them carefully in the hall.

That evening I was telling my husband, George, about the disheartening chore and was commenting on the scandalous waste of fine furniture. I was particularly upset about a beautiful dining table and matching set of chairs, which would have been an ideal replacement for the battered furniture we'd had since our marriage.

'Dealers will get them', said George, cynically. 'Sharks who'll pick them up for a song and make a packet.'

I felt it was criminal for those lovely pieces to go to strangers with no feeling for their loving history. George suggested that we offered to buy them. It would hardly matter to Lily; she might even be pleased if they went to someone who appreciated her fine things. I explained that a solicitor working for the Court of Protection was dealing with her effects, but George scoffed.

Lily, he pointed out, was sitting on a fortune. Her vast house and grounds would be snapped up by developers, so a few paltry bits of furniture were inconsequential. Besides, he added, from what he knew of my clients, she would barely know what was happening. It seemed an unrepeatable opportunity for us, and of course we would pay; there was no question of dishonesty, and Lily would not be deprived.

On my next visit to Lily I stated my interest in buying her antique table, eight matching chairs, a chest of drawers and a handsome potstand. I was surprised that she understood about the proceedings with her solicitor, and when she said that all the furniture had to go to the salerooms, I assured her that it wouldn't matter if she sold a few pieces beforehand.

She hesitated and I said, 'Why let indifferent merchants handle your precious furniture, when I would really care for it? Besides, who would know?' Lily mentioned a price, but I didn't want to pay that much.

I left and 'phoned later, offering her the lesser sum of £140 for the lot, reminding her that a dealer might only take it for scrap. Eventually Lily conceded, saying, 'Oh well, Kathleen, as it is *you*. . .'

The old lady was due to move on Tuesday morning and the auctioneers would collect the remaining furniture that afternoon, so we had to act quickly. George borrowed a van on Monday, and I arranged for Mark to accompany my husband, to direct the way to Lily's house and give a hand lifting the known objects. As I had just drawn the money from my bank, I asked Mark to hand £100 to Lily, and sent him later with the outstanding £40.

Much to my surprise, two weeks after this transaction, I was called to my director of nursing services, to speak about some missing furniture. I guessed that meddling Phyllis was at the bottom of all this. The social worker was jealous of my closeness with the clients, and was now trying to make life difficult for me.

My conscience was perfectly clear, but I wanted to avoid unnecessary embarrassment and bad publicity for the centre. So I had a word with young Mark, asking if he might say that I had lent him the money to buy the furniture for his needy parents. Unfortunately he was not as willing as I had presumed. He flatly refused to uphold a false story and promptly revealed the truth to the DNS.

I denied that I had been in breach of my professional Code. Lily had been satisfied with the deal and had agreed to the exchange. My client had not suffered a loss and, after all, the items had been for sale. I do not know what all the fuss is about. **"**

The official decision, and discussion

Part 1 of the Code of Professional Conduct states that, 'Each registered nurse, midwife and health visitor, in the exercise of professional accountability, shall act always in such a way as to promote and safeguard the well being and interests of patients/clients.'

Part 8 of the Code states, 'Each registered nurse [etc] shall avoid any abuse of the privileged relationship which exists with patients/clients and of the privileged access allowed to their property, residence or place of work.'

In an interview with the DNS, this nurse made it clear that she understood the role of the Court of Protection and that this meant the patient was incapable of managing her own affairs, particularly concerning finances. Kathleen had known it was wrong to deal directly with the client, but had made no attempt to approach the solicitor. Clearly, she was taking advantage of her position and contravening clauses 1 and 8 of the Code.

The client might have been unusual in being the subject of Court of Protection orders. Although she was regarded as able to live alone up until the move, she was deemed incapable of managing her financial affairs, and it was in this respect that particular advantage was taken of her. The items which Kathleen acquired were of far greater value than the sum she paid.

The Committee particularly disliked the way in which the

young community worker was made use of. Although recruited through social services, he spent much of his time working at the centre with the nurses or going with them on visits. The event involving the exchange of furniture for money happened early in his employment and, with no previous knowledge of the work, he considered it logical to follow the nurse's instructions about moving furniture and handing over the money.

When Kathleen subsequently tried to get him to falsify the account, and implicate himself as dishonest, he refused to be a party to the fabrication of an untrue story.

The decision of the Committee was to remove this nurse from the professional Register.

The final straw

It is difficult to maintain professional standards within a setting where staff complacency conspires to sanction unsatisfactory care. The individual who attempts to question from within a system that has deteriorated is a lone voice, a dissenter, who meets a barrier of inaction, disregard, scorn, even hostility. Alienated, surrounded by apathy, yet powerless to change things, the conscientious practitioner has a fruitless struggle to uphold personal standards. In the end, individual effort may not survive collective abrogation of responsibility.

❝ I am deeply committed to working with people with a mental handicap. I thoroughly enjoy being an enrolled nurse and I feel I have a lot to offer. Naturally there are moments of frustration, but working with handicapped people has many joys and rewards.

During my training we were highly motivated and encouraged; having the support of enthusiastic and innovative teaching staff helped the learners and kept interest alive among permanent staff.

I took my ideals and aspirations to my new post at St Margaret's. In this cottage unit with two bungalows for 24 residents with varying degrees of handicap, I was confronted by demoralised staff who had lost all interest. They made little attempt to improve the lives of their clients and, perhaps more worrying, were disinclined to let anyone else try.

It was an apathetic, sterile environment, where staff were content to keep the status quo and no one wanted to rock the boat. They condoned the lowest denominator of care; a repetitive series of basic life sustaining tasks was the limit of their involvement.

Every day the same routine was followed – getting everybody up, to the bathroom, then to the dining room for breakfast. In a hectic rush each resident was bathed, dressed and toiletted as quickly as possible. Speed and efficiency were crucial. The unit's routine was regimented and largely inflexible, with little or no margin for residents' personal choice.

This tightly structured arrangement did not match my experience of good care. I found it difficult to do my job properly and to maintain a high standard of nursing, which would have meant working slower, at the residents' pace, to help them achieve goals of personal care. But when other staff worked quickly, 'getting more done', they complained that I was not pulling my weight.

Finding a balance between what was best for the residents and managing to get everything done was extremely difficult, and ultimately it was our clients that suffered.

New staff would arrive full of enthusiasm and good ideas,

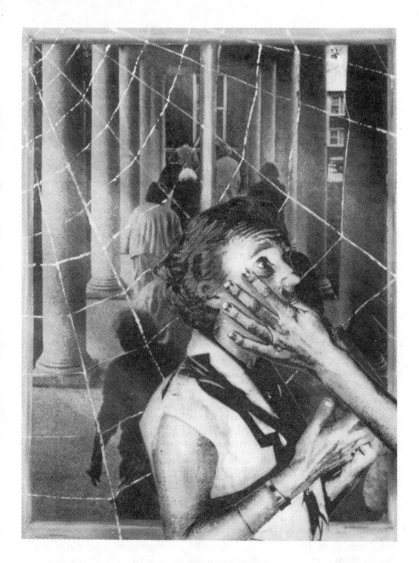

recognising the wretched situation and keen to breathe life back into the unit. Faced with an unsupported uphill struggle, they soon became disillusioned or cynical, like the rest of the nurses.

Any suggestions for change were treated with suspicion, from the sister down to the nursing assistants, because of extra work that might be involved. They were also regarded as veiled, and unwelcome, criticism.

Two learners did go to the sister to request that only one resident should be in the bathroom at a time. This change was agreed and, although it meant more work, it was an improvement and gave the residents some dignity. I was fairly certain, however, that the sister, staff nurse and I were the only ones to abide by this, as other staff needed constant reminders. Limited bathing and toilet facilities were a good excuse for taking short cuts.

Mealtimes were total chaos. We rarely had more than three or four staff on duty. One room was for more able residents, who could be supervised by domestics and housekeepers, which left the nurses free to cope with those who needed assistance.

Sharing three or four staff for 10 people who all needed some supervision – anything from prompting to complete feeding – was very difficult. It became a refuelling exercise on a conveyor belt, devoid of enjoyment or social interaction – and it made me squirm.

The whole situation was a nightmare and I felt powerless to do anything about it. Who could I tell? The sister seemed impervious to comments or suggestions. She had previously worked at a children's unit and treated adult residents in the same way.

She was opposed to letting the residents have alcohol, although the strongest they drank was a half pint or two of shandy. She did not allow them to have more than 50 pence to go out with, even at Christmas. She was reluctant to hold staff meetings, even though there had been repeated requests for this.

What good would it do to take my complaints higher? Telling tales about well meaning, but overworked, demoralised colleagues did not appeal to me. I just hoped that the imminent arrival of a new director of nursing might improve things.

On his first day in office we had only two staff on duty for 24 residents and could get no help from other units, not even for a few hours. I was deeply concerned for the welfare of the residents and decided to ring the trade union representative. Within 15 minutes help had arrived. The following day the new nursing officer wanted to know who had caused *trouble* by contacting and involving the union!

During the year I worked in the cottage unit I became increasingly disgusted with myself, my colleagues and the system. We gave our residents only the absolute basics of nursing care, and even that ineffectually. It was a soul destroying experience.

One particular day I was especially worried about Angela who looked as though she had given up and wanted to die. She was eating and drinking very little, and showed no interest in anything. My anger and frustration were intense because I felt that our rotten system had made her that way. The residents had nothing to live for, no enjoyment, no motivation and no dignity. They walked around in disgraceful clothes that looked as if they came straight from a jumble sale, and anything sent to the launderette came back ruined.

When the staff nurse on duty with me went for tea, I thought I would try to cheer up Angela with a chocolate drink. Just then, Michael, who is prone to aggressive outbursts, came towards me, kicked out and slapped me; then he spat in my face.

I stood motionless. Policy dictates that a nurse should walk away and not get involved in a confrontation. But how could I stand back when I saw that Michael was about to lash out at Angela, too? I saw the fear in her eyes and became angry. This was the final straw. Without a second thought, I went towards him and, as he raised his leg, hit him smartly on the thigh, as the only immediate means to protect the girl.

Afterwards, I was sick and disgusted at what I had done, even though it was the result of extreme provocation and I had tried to help another resident. I knew I had acted wrongly, but I could not bring myself to tell anyone. No one had witnessed the incident, yet my conscience was troubling me and I had difficulty sleeping.

There seemed to be no one to turn to and, as far as I knew, there was no procedure to cover such a situation. Eventually I summoned up courage and confessed to the nursing officer that I had struck one of the residents. It was actually a relief to be able to tell someone, and I accepted that my action had contravened the Code of Professional Conduct.

I very much regret what took place. In a way it was a cry for help for myself and the people I look after, who deserve good professional care. I felt trapped in a web of difficult circumstances beyond my control.

I hope that this incident will bring about some changes to benefit residents and staff. It should not be swept under the carpet and forgotten, as has been the case up to now. **"**

Think points

- Which parts of the Code are under question here?
- List the factors which contribute to a lowering of standards of nursing care.
- Discuss the factors which bring about lack of interest and low morale in nursing staff.
- What may dissuade a nurse from making a complaint to her superiors?
- Using personal examples, discuss how the actions and attitudes of other members of a nursing team have influenced your performance, for better and for worse.
- Can you suggest any other people in whom this nurse could have confided her anxieties?
- Using your judgement, do you consider that she should be accused of professional misconduct?

The official decision, and discussion

Part 1 of the Code of Professional Conduct states that, 'Each registered nurse, midwife and health visitor is accountable for his or her practice and in the exercise of professional accountability shall act always in such a way as to promote and safeguard the well being and interests of patients/clients.'

Part 10 of the Code states that, 'Each registered nurse [etc] shall have regard to the environment of care and its physical, psychological and social effects on patients/clients, and also to the adequacy of resources, and make known to appropriate persons or authorities any circumstances which could place patients/clients in jeopardy or which militate against safe standards of practice.'

From the evidence received, the Committee felt this young woman was clearly a kind, competent and caring nurse, ideally suited to the care of people with a mental handicap. The fact that she cared so much made her vulnerable when working in a setting which made it extremely difficult for her to practise safely and well.

The nurse's account of her difficulties illustrates the problems of delivering good care, irrespective of the specialty.

The Committee was particularly aware that, had the nurse herself not told others that she had slapped a resident, no one would ever have known.

It was also noted that she was not able to withdraw from the situation, as the policy on violent incidents would have had her do, since that would have left a weaker resident at serious risk of harm.

In view of all the circumstances, although the slapping of a patient is regarded as misconduct, the Committee placed this incident very low on the scale of such offences and took no action.

Criticism was addressed to the managers of St Margaret's and its future as a training hospital was put under review.

The buck stops here

All too often, nurses will blindly follow doctors' instructions in the belief that they must be correct and that their medical colleagues will take responsibility for errors. Both assumptions are false, and nurses are held to be accountable for their own professional performance.

66 I met Hilary Compton in the corridor as I made my way to work for the night shift. Hilary, sister in charge of the four medical wards, checked her duty sheet anxiously and said she was pleased that I was covering the busy female ward.

'You've got auxiliary nurse Chin; I'm sorry I can't give you any more help but there is no one else available,' she said.

One staff nurse and an untrained helper to care for the total needs of 28 patients was the prospect that faced us. The patients included many elderly ladies, heavy, immobile and incontinent, who would keep us busy throughout the night. I was pleased to be allocated Molly Chin, a marvellous auxiliary who knew the ward well. As Hilary had optimistically forecast, I had no doubt that we would 'manage OK'.

'Managing', 'coping' and 'muddling through' were familiar to us – they had become almost a way of life. Hilary and I, each with 25 years' experience, often discussed the diabolical lack of resources on the unit.

The situation had become so worrying the previous Christmas that we compiled a report which we signed and sent to the director of nursing services. Taking one typical night, we made a detailed list of the 130 patients in the unit, their problems, level of dependence and nursing requirements. This was matched to staffing allocation in order to demonstrate the inadequate and, frankly, dangerous level of cover.

We also pointed out that nurses were not prepared to work in such stressful conditions, that they were leaving in droves and that it was impossible to recruit replacements.

Our carefully prepared document was not well received by the director of nursing services. We were fobbed off with the usual excuses about stretched finances and management constraints. Our comments had been 'duly noted' and that was the last we heard of it. This was not much solace to us, struggling at the bedside, watching helplessly as standards of care inevitably fell, but at least we had registered our protest.

That Sunday night Molly and I concentrated on getting the patients settled quickly, as there were several who would need attention to nasogastric feeding and intravenous lines, routine observations and preparation for investigations the following day.

Sister from the accident department rang to confirm that we had a spare bed. She wanted to admit a young woman who, because of postnatal depression, had swallowed nearly a whole bottle of paracetamol tablets. As a precaution, A&E had done a stomach washout but, believing that Mrs Styles had ingested these pills at lunchtime, almost 12 hours before, it was imperative that she had an antidote infusion set up immediately she was settled in the ward.

I suggested that she would be better suited to ICU, where I knew they had beds, staff and the correct facilities to offer such critical care. Dr Roberts insisted that the patient should come to my ward. Hilary explained that we were short of nurses and that admitting Mrs Styles would dilute care to the existing patients.

None of this concerned the admitting doctor. He did not think it appropriate for an unhappy woman to be put into ICU because he thought she was not too ill and the environment might disturb her.

We put Mrs Styles in a bed close to the nurses' station and helped get an infusion established. Dr Roberts consulted his pocket book to work out that a woman weighing 60 kg needed 9000 mg of Parvolex by slow infusion.

It was not a drug I was familiar with, so while the doctor wrote it up, Hilary and I searched the stock cupboard. I eventually handed Dr Roberts a box of eight ampoules. He took one, read '200 mg' and did some speedy calculations.

'My God, is this all you have?' he snapped. 'There isn't sufficient here to treat a mouse! She'll need 45 ampoules. I'll fetch some more while you draw these up.'

Hilary and I agreed that 45 ampoules of 10 ml sounded an enormous amount of fluid to add to the intravenous bags. Just then Molly Chin told us that Miss Simmonds was having breathing difficulties, Miss Hazel in her demented state was 'off to catch the bus home' and Mrs Turner in the side ward had disconnected her catheter and soaked the bed.

Hilary said she would give Molly a hand if I could continue preparing the intravenous bags. None of us had had a meal break, not even a cup of tea, and it didn't look as if we would for a while.

Dr Roberts returned with an armful of Parvolex boxes which he put in the treatment room. He quickly checked that the prescription was in order and that Mrs Styles' drip was running satisfactorily, while I answered his bleep. He was called to another crisis in A&E and dashed off, leaving us to sort out the drip.

Our hectic schedule continued throughout the night. It was rewarding that Mrs Styles seemed happy to be alive and was speaking positively about her baby. We assured her that, once the antidote had done its work and the drug was cleared from her system, she and her daughter would be reunited.

Regrettably, this was not to be. By early morning, when Mrs Styles' infusion was almost completed, she developed disturbing symptoms indicating that all was not well. She was extremely pale, had abdominal cramps, was delerious, had a poor urinary output, low blood pressure and an erratic pulse. Dr Roberts discontinued the remainder of the Parvolex infusion and arranged for her to be transferred immediately to ICU, although her deterioration was a puzzle to everyone.

As the nurse responsible for the handover to ICU staff, I explained about Mrs Styles' nursing care and mentioned casually that a large volume of the antidote solution had been needed. The ICU sister could not understand this and, when I checked an ampoule, I found to my horror that there had been a ten-fold error in the estimations. The ampoule stated, although not very clearly, 200 mg per ml in each 10 ml ampoule – not 200 mg per ampoule, as we had believed.

In retrospect, it was blindingly obvious that Hilary or I should have double checked the drug. But because of the overwhelming demands on our time, we had foolishly accepted the doctor's estimation without question.

The mistake was found too late to be of any help to Mrs Styles, who died the following day.

Her death was the subject of a coroner's inquest, which Hilary, I and Dr Roberts had to attend. The pathologist was unable to state the precise cause of death; obviously a substantial overdose of Parvolex was implicated but the massive ingestion of paracetamol could equally have been to blame. There was no way of telling conclusively and no guilt was attributed.

This made it all the more surprising when Hilary and I were made the subjects of complaint by our health authority and brought before a Professional Conduct Committee hearing. I didn't think they had a case against us. After all, we had been saying for months that we were working under tremendous pressure, that we were short of staff and resources in a busy unit. And we had documented evidence to support these claims.

The error was a classic one. Even the coroner misread the drug ampoule and box when shown the evidence. The doctor made the initial mistake and compounded it by his subsequent actions. Although his prescription was accurate, his interpretation was not, and we were aggrieved that the authority did not mete out the same treatment to the medical staff as it did to us nurses. **99**

The official decision, and discussion

Part 4 of the Code of Professional Conduct states that, 'Each registered nurse, midwife and health visitor is accountable for his or her practice, and, in the exercise of professional accountability shall acknowledge any limitations of competence and refuse in such cases to accept delegated functions without first having received instruction in regard to those functions and having been assessed as competent.'

At a joint hearing, the Committee was faced with two experienced, conscientious and effective nurses with exemplary career records. They had been striving to do their best in difficult circumstances, working under continuous pressure for a substantial period of time. As the Code of Professional Conduct requests, they had drawn attention to their managers of the dangers at work, initially by letter and then with a lengthy and comprehensive document.

This document was of particular significance, for a great deal of the respondents' time and effort had been taken to apply their considerable experience, resulting in a dossier which clearly demonstrated the large gap between needs and resources. It was reprehensible that they received a brush-off from the managers, with an unsympathetic and unhelpful reply.

The Committee considered the background to the tragic event and the submission by lawyers on behalf of the two nurses, which challenged the allegation of misconduct.

In conclusion, the admitted facts were not regarded as misconduct in view of the appalling context within which the unfortunate incident occurred. The managers were publicly criticised.

It was also noted that, once again, nurses had been brought before a disciplinary hearing while the doctor was not the subject of a complaint to his regulating body. Medical staff are advised not to get involved in UKCC hearings or assist in the defence of professional colleagues.

This case is a salutory reminder 'only to act if you are convinced that it is safe to do so'.

Sleeping on the job

It is well known and easy to understand how work related anxieties can tumble over into personal life, with varying effects. However, what of the consequences when personal crisis and domestic difficulties encroach on professional performance, to compromise standards of care? It is implicit in the trained nurse's role that she has continued responsibility for the patients in her care, required to be constantly vigilant and attentive to their needs. This story also clearly illustrates that for registration status to be held in question, a mistake or accident need not necessarily occur.

❝ Because Larkton Manor Hospital is a sprawling estate of widely placed units, it has the notable disadvantage of making night supervision difficult and laborious.

The area mainly affected is the acute admission wards, which are conveniently clustered around the administration block. Patients here exhibit disturbed, aggressive or suicidal behaviour and consequently need constant close attention.

It is, therefore, particularly fortunate that I can usually count on the rest of the hospital remaining quiet. The continuing care units house the chronically mentally ill, the frail elderly and the 'burnt out' schizophrenics, whose agitation has been dampened, whose personalities have been damaged by their illness and whose behaviour has been moulded by institutionalisation.

These units are in the peaceful, remote outskirts of the estate, forming part of the rehabilitation complex. It is easy to see why they are called 'back wards'.

I have always been confident that I can rely on our regular team of night nurses, who are familiar with the routine and understand their patients. Many of these staff have been at Larkton Manor for a number of years in the same unchanging role. It is cruel to suggest that the nurses are as institutionalised as the patients but, with recruitment difficulties in our area, we are thankful for these reliable people who are loyal to the hospital.

There is only one nurse allocated to each ward because the patients are subdued and behave in predictable and automatic ways. Things are improving slowly but it is unrealistic to expect the lone night nurse to continue much of the rehabilitation programme on his shift.

The evening routine is much the same in all the long stay wards. A group of patients watch television and the nurse would give the smokers a final cigarette and supervise them being lit. He would then, perhaps, play a game of snooker with one of the patients, while a couple of others gave out the night drinks and washed up.

After dishing out the night medication and ensuring that each patient had been to the toilet, the nurse would encourage the last of the stragglers to bed.

On the whole, a nurse could be assured of an undisturbed night and, although it was accepted that night nurses might find it difficult not to doze occasionally in the chair, outright sleeping was forbidden. One staff member was recently dismissed for moonlighting in the day and catching up on his sleep during night duty.

Admittedly it is not a taxing job but each nurse is responsible for the 30 or more dependent people who, for security and safety, must be locked in at night. The variety of potential risks is frightening and emphasises the need for constant vigilance; the hazards from fire, electrical appliances, illicit smoking in bed, gas in the kitchen, potent drugs in stock, sudden illness or violent outbursts.

My first task that Sunday night was to check each ward, staffing levels and inpatient lists. I knew all the patients by name on Darwin Ward and was happy to note that Jim Croker, an enrolled nurse, was in charge that night. An exceptionally pleasant young man, Jim had moved into the area when he married and had been a good nurse during his six years with us.

For a while I had to help out in the female acute ward, which was having one of those memorably chaotic evenings familiar to any psychiatric nurse. Having completed the incident form on a girl who had cut her wrists, it was time for my second tour of the hospital.

The rehabilitation complex was peaceful, as expected. Jim's patients were settled and sleeping, so he was in the office with a coffee and several newspapers. He was efficient and polite but not one for social chatter and he revealed little about himself.

Over the weekend I had twisted my ankle and now, after two long treks around the hospital, it was starting to throb and was visibly swollen. Feeling satisfied that the wards were tranquil and well staffed, I decided against making a third round, which I normally did around 4 am.

Instead, I telephoned the wards to check that all was well. However, I could not get an answer from Darwin Ward, although I tried twice. Perhaps Jim was involved with one of the old men who needed help getting to the toilet, or perhaps someone was confused. There were as many possible reasons why he did not answer as there were patients. Then my bleep went.

I was called to the male acute ward, where a young man was being admitted exhibiting frank, bizarre persecutory delusions. He was accompanied by his worried, bewildered and tearful parents and we reassured them about their son.

I presumed that Jim Croker had considered it too dangerous to leave a patient unattended while he ran to answer the telephone. I could not have been more wrong!

Unbeknown to anyone, Jim had been involved in some bitter domestic problems in previous months, which erupted in a crisis that Sunday afternoon. I was not aware of any difficulties, neither did I notice any change in his quiet, reserved behaviour.

Jim had brought a bottle of vodka to work, perhaps because it has virtually no odour and can be drunk without arousing suspicion.

Once the patients had settled to sleep and I was safely out of view just after midnight, Jim made a start on the bottle and finished it during the next two hours. At first he was relaxed and happier than he had been for ages. Then he had difficulty keeping his eyes open.

Making his way back unsteadily from the toilet, Jim met one of his patients. 'You look tired Jim,' he said. 'You ought to have a lie down for a while, why don't you go to bed?'

Jim recognised it as a good suggestion and staggered along the dimly lit dormitory and gratefully took to a bed where, for four hours, he remained oblivious to his surroundings.

At 6.45 am, nearing the end of that night shift, I telephoned Elliot Ward to ask if their second nurse would kindly collect all the night reports for me from the rehabilitation complex. This student arrived at Darwin Ward as the day sister turned up for her 7 am start. The telephone rang and the day sister answered a caller who wanted to speak to Jim Croker. The student and Sister, therefore, went looking for Jim, without success.

A helpful patient asked if they were looking for the night nurse and, when told they were, said, 'He's down there in bed.'

Much to their amazement, the student and Sister found Jim sharing an occupied bed, with the legitimate occupant looking like a bird whose nest had been invaded by a snoring, slumbering cuckoo. Appreciating the delicacy of the situation, Sister first made sure that the patient was not unduly distressed. The old man said he didn't mind very much but added that he found the bed a bit narrow for two!

Jim was so deeply asleep that the sister had to shout loudly and shake him vigorously in order to rouse him. Once Jim woke and moved to get out of the bed, the two nurses realised that he was wearing only his underpants. So astonished was she, the sister simply told Jim that he was wanted on the telephone. In retrospect, this was facile and wholly inappropriate, considering the gravity of the situation, and provided an unintended note of humour when recounted at the subsequent UKCC hearing.

The incident was reported to the director of nursing services, who intended to contact Jim later in the day, to advise him of his immediate suspension from duty pending further inquiries. However, before this could happen, Jim returned to the hospital and insisted on speaking to the DNS. He was warned not to say anything self incriminating and was advised to be accompanied for the interview, so that an observer could witness the conversation.

But without waiting for a representative, Jim simply blurted out that he drank on duty because of personal pressures and he agreed with the account given by the other members of staff. Although he admitted that it had been unwise to go to bed, he believed it to be unoccupied at the time. Having got this off his chest, he **99** handed over his written resignation and left the hospital.

Think points

- Which parts of the Code are under question here?
- What factors may have influenced this nurse's decision to risk bringing alcohol to work and contributed to a heavy drinking session?
- List the dangers which could befall a group of elderly patients with chronic mental and physical disabilities, when locked in a ward without supervision.
- Can you suggest avenues of help available to a nurse who needs advice or counselling with personal problems?
- Discuss the ways in which personal difficulties may manifest themselves in someone's work performance.
- Using your judgement, do you consider this nurse could be accused of professional misconduct?

The official decision, and discussion

Part 1 of the Code of Professional Conduct states that, 'Each registered nurse, midwife and health visitor is accountable for his or her practice, and in the exercise of professional accountability shall act always in such a way as to promote and safeguard the well being and interests of patients/ clients.'

Part 2 of the Code states that, 'Each registered nurse [etc] shall ensure that no action or omission on his/her part or within his/ her sphere of influence is detrimental to the condition or safety of patients/clients.'

Jim Croker was the subject of charges before a Professional Conduct Committee hearing, with allegations on two counts, of drinking alcohol on duty and sleeping in a patient's bed. Although he had been served formal notice of the hearing to his registered address, Jim had neither sent a statement or explanation for the Investigating Committee, nor did he attend the hearing. The Committee, therefore, had no direct evidence from the respondent. They had to assess his case on the evidence of the three prime witnesses, whose statements corroborated the facts above.

The decision of the Committee was to remove Jim from the professional Register.

Dangerous pride

Nothing is more dangerous than the jealous guarding of professional autonomy. Practitioners must appreciate their own boundaries and limitations, while respecting those of others. Working in a multidisciplinary system means dovetailing with other professionals and making use of the available services to ensure the best patient care. There is no virtue in struggling on blindly alone, racked with indecision and hesitation that may cause a fatal delay. Certainly there is no professional disgrace in seeking advice and help from others. Although midwives are governed by some different rules, this story is useful to illustrate the need to work in co-operation with other professional staff.

66 It was my duty evening on call, covering for the community midwifery service. Having visited each of my clients, I knew all was well on my patch.

After a tiring day I'd taken a warm, soothing bath before settling down to eat my supper in front of the TV. But my favourite serial was interrupted by a phone call from the hospital emergency bed service which forwards urgent messages to the duty midwife.

It concerned a young girl who had delivered her first baby nine days ago. Out of the blue she had started to bleed and this continued steadily for several hours – now she was losing blood clots. This dramatic scene was painted by her agitated boyfriend. Judging by the tone of the message, I wondered if the situation had been exaggerated through anxiety and ignorance. I daresay they were worrying unnecessarily.

I finished my meal, got dressed and reached the family about an hour later. They lived in a poky flat on a rundown council estate.

A spotty youth, polite enough, answered the door and led me through the dingy hall to the room where his girlfriend lay in bed. I quickly assessed the situation, and immediately complained about the inconveniently low divan. I have chronic back pain which is not helped by having to bend and crouch.

I read the co-operative card. Tracy, the 16-year old mother, lived with Darren, the 18-year old father of the baby. There had been an uneventful pregnancy, normal delivery and puerperium. The baby was well cared for; the mother was not breastfeeding and there had been no problems until she began to bleed vaginally.

Tracy had noticed a slight blood loss that afternoon and, uncertain what it meant, stayed in bed until her boyfriend came home. Darren left her to rest while he prepared their meal and fed the baby. He appeared to be a sensible, practical lad and fond of his child.

Later Tracy needed to go to the toilet but as she rose from the bed

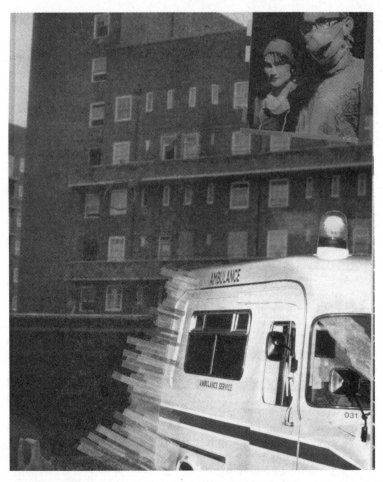

she was horrified to see a huge blood clot fall onto the rug. She said it was the size of an orange, although I assured her that congealed blood looks deceptively large. During the subsequent hour large clots came with increasing frequency.

Darren did not know what he should do but had the presence of mind to gather up the clots and store them in plastic bin liners. He showed me the collection neatly stacked in the bath. Eventually Darren had left Tracy while he searched for a telephone box that had not been vandalised.

The girl looked pale, but then the sight of blood upsets many people. I struggled to kneel in order to examine her. She was a tubby girl with a 'floppy' postnatal abdomen, so I prodded gently to palpate the uterus. I thought it a bit 'boggy' but not sufficiently so to warrant a postpartum haemorrhage. In the meantime, Darren was answering the door to visitors who were popping in every five minutes. Family and friends gathered in the kitchen when they knew I was examining Tracy.

Darren helped me put an incontinence pad under Tracy and I left a few spares for later use. With difficulty, I stood up and instructed him to continue saving the clots and clearing up the leaky mess. But first I asked him to bring me a chair, so that I could sit comfortably and write my notes.

I was thinking out loud and deciding whether or not I should call an ambulance. If Tracy was having a haemorrhage this would certainly be necessary but, as this was not the situation at present, further interference was not warranted. Not being *utterly* certain, I didn't want to confuse or alarm the young parents so I said nothing definite and hastily left the flat. I felt sure they could cope now, having other helpers at hand to offer support.

I drove to the local hospital to make further enquiries in a roundabout way. In the obstetric unit, where I was well known, I saw the labour suite sister at her desk, completing the diary notes ready for the night staff. I struck up a casual conversation about circumstances relating to postpartum haemorrhage and we discussed various hypothetical questions.

I decided to cover myself by telephoning the patient's GP to put him in the picture. Quite incidentally, I checked with him at what degree of severity he might consider it necessary to mobilise help and which of the emergency services might be appropriate. Not, of course, that it was relevant, for I was on my way back to see the patient shortly.

As I approached the estate I noticed the flashing blue light of an ambulance parked close to Tracy's block of flats. Rushing in, I was pushed aside rudely by two ambulance men attempting to remove Tracy on a stretcher. 'Kindly stand back, move out of our way, madam, this patient needs *urgent* hospital attention without further delay,' one of them said. In that curt remark I sensed hostility and felt offended that my responsibility and authority had been undermined. Darren accompanied Tracy in the ambulance while I remained in the flat.

The family were not at all welcoming but greeted the GP warmly when he arrived, minutes after Tracy had been rushed away. Tracy's mother explained what had happened. During my absence the family had taken their cue from Darren's sister, coincidentally also in the late stages of pregnancy. Barbara, who was a nurse and midwife, although currently not working, had gone to see Tracy after I left. She was disturbed to hear of the bleeding and shocked to see the evidence of considerable blood loss. Not having the kind of drugs that I carry, her only recourse was to attempt to 'rub up' a contraction.

Barbara urged the relatives to call an ambulance, but initially they resisted, not wishing to upset me, as they felt I might have been on my way for help. As Tracy's condition deteriorated, Barbara vehemently insisted that an ambulance be called.

Tracy's mother complained to the GP that her daughter had been left 'bleeding to death', with no explanation and no offer of help from me, and described how they had finally acted in desperation to call for emergency help.

The doctor looked in amazement at the collection of plastic bags containing clots and the blood-soaked linen and pads. He drove directly to the hospital to report his findings. I could only believe that Tracy's condition must have worsened since I originally left the flat. It would have been impossible to predict that she could have deteriorated so suddenly.

In the A&E department Tracy had already been seen by the casualty officer, who had taken blood for cross-matching and instantly set up an IV infusion. When the obstetric senior registrar was called to take over the case, he said it was the worst postpartum haemorrhage he had ever witnessed, which seemed a bit of an exaggeration to me. Tracy was whisked into theatre for an urgent evacuation of retained products of conception and following a transfusion of three units of blood, she made a satisfactory recovery.

My management of this case was questioned and I became the subject of a misconduct hearing alleging a sequence of failures to take appropriate action. I agreed that the events happened but did not agree with the accusations that I had failed as a midwife. Certainly this would have been true if my patient had been having a postpartum haemorrhage, but in my judgement, based on years of experience, this was not so.

Think points

- Which part of the Code is under question here?
- Discuss reasons why a nurse, midwife or health visitor may resist calling another professional for assistance.
- Discuss the value of listening to patients and relatives in assessing their situation. Give examples from your own practice.
- Discuss the influence of cultural factors and value judgements affecting patient care.
- Consider the positive and negative aspects of a practitioner described as 'experienced with longstanding service'.
- What guidance points could you give to senior student nurses concerning their responsibility to alert other professional help?
- Do you consider this midwife guilty of professional misconduct?

The official decision, and discussion

Part 5 of the Code of Professional Conduct states that, 'Each registered nurse, midwife and health visitor is accountable for his or her practice and, in the exercise of professional accountability, shall work in a collaborative and co-operative manner with other health care professionals and recognise and respect their particular contributions within the health care team.'

The witnesses in this case unanimously verified that the patient was the victim of a severe postpartum haemorrhage, which justified early, prompt treatment and required making use of the emergency services available.

The labour suite sister in the obstetric unit knew her colleague to be an experienced and long-serving community midwife and was surprised that she was asking questions about when you would call the obstetric flying squad or an ambulance with IV infusion equipment. It never occurred to the sister that the community midwife was alluding to a *real* patient.

The GP had been rather confused after the midwife's telephone call. Although she had not requested a visit, the doctor was sufficiently concerned to decide it would be safer to see the patient for himself. He found evidence of severe, sustained and prolonged vaginal bleeding, indicative of a critical postpartum haemorrhage. Both the casualty officer and senior registrar confirmed that Tracy was seriously ill on admission to A&E and that it had been fortunate that her sister-in-law had intervened swiftly.

The respondent continued to insist that it had not been a postpartum haemorrhage but offered no alternative that could explain such a significant blood loss over several hours. She was unmoved by the evidence of the three doctors involved.

The Committee found the midwife guilty of professional misconduct and removed her name from the Register.

An expensive claim

Honesty and integrity are implicit in the role of the professional nurse and responsible behaviour must be upheld if autonomous practice is safely to be assured. There are numerous opportunities for corruption and theft within the health system, while individual claims may arouse suspicion.

66 Sometimes my managers must think there are eight days to a week, judging by the way work is heaped onto my caseload. After all, there is a limit to the number of visits a district nurse can reasonably be expected to squeeze into a normal working day.

I am not a dawdler but I believe it is important to give each client personal attention and commitment when I call at his home. I try to offer a caring service, considerate of individual circumstances, while always being a safe practitioner.

During my 12 years at this health practice I have enjoyed good working relations with all my colleagues – nurses, doctors, other professionals and support staff. I am generally allocated patients from the lists of the two senior GPs, with whom I have developed a good rapport. I understand their clinical preferences, attitudes and approaches – their 'little ways'.

It is obviously good to have close teamwork and continuity of service, which enables me to get to know clients and their families well. This contributes to better care and adds to my job satisfaction. One slight drawback is the wide geographical spread of clients, which necessitates a considerable amount of travelling, crisscrossing the borough as needs demand.

Like many community staff, I have a Crown car and have taken advantage of the concession which allows me private use of it if I pay a monthly fee and a mileage charge. This perk saves our family the considerable expense of having to buy a second car for me. We use my husband's car for long distance holiday and day trips, while I tend to reserve my work car for small local journeys.

Community staff complete monthly travel returns, submitted to the district transport officer, who makes the final calculations, and authorises any charges to be deducted from our salary. We do not have an outlay for petrol at source, because we fill up our cars at garages which have a direct arrangement with the health authority.

The whole system works well, although I think we all agree that filling in the necessary forms is tedious and time consuming. I usually do it 'by the book', starting the trip counter at nought each morning, then charting the number of miles covered by the end of every day.

Last summer we were unexpectedly stretched for nursing cover on the district, with not only normal holiday leave, but one sister on extended sickness and my best enrolled nurse having moved out of the area. At the same time, Dr Trent was anxious that we provide better team support for families who wanted to care for their terminally ill relatives at home.

My work was heavy and demanding, physically and emotionally; I was being pulled in all directions to juggle with the priorities from every corner of the neighbourhood. I was also responsible for learners on their community allocation and for a district nursing student on placement, whose caseload I had to supervise.

A day's record of visits never accurately reflected the extent of my duties; things were not as straightforward as might have appeared from my diary. I made all the calls indicated but not necessarily in the order shown, nor to the best geographical sequence. Timed calls always took priority, such as injections of morphia or insulin, and some patients required more than one visit a day. I would also have to meet set appointments during my rounds; to catch the GPs in surgery hours, hold a clinic at the health centre, collect dressings or prescriptions, or join the team for a planned home visit for a patient due to be discharged from hospital.

In my off duty lunch hour, I might pop into the shops, the library, or visit the dentist – I would deduct the miles to account for this personal car use. However, it was such a busy time for me, I knew I wasn't making many private journeys.

I was behind with my book-keeping, although my diary remained my 'bible' for a daily action plan and record of visits. I got out of the habit of logging my mileage each day, finding that I had to complete the whole of the preceding month's travel returns by referring to my diary. I continued to take the cumulative total at the end of one month to be the starting figure for the subsequent month and worked out the mileage without even referring to the car's mileometer.

I found I cut through the paperwork with this simple, straightforward and efficient method. As I did about the same number of miles each month, it looked plausible on paper, so I decided to stick to this approach, not worrying unduly about the petty forms, thus allowing more valuable time to concentrate on patient care.

Towards Christmas, the car was difficult to start so I took it to the transport officer for a check. After two days I was called to see my nursing officer, who questioned me about my travel returns, explaining that the transport officer had brought a discrepancy to her attention.

By coincidence, the transport officer had been checking the claim forms of all the cars in the fleet, to plan the priorities for servicing and mine had not been due to be called in. But when he looked at my car's mileometer, he noticed that it was registering nearly 10 000 miles – showing that servicing was necessary.

The transport officer tried, without success, to find an error on my claim forms that would account for the extra 1500 miles used on the car. When he could not, he was duty bound to report the discrepancy to my nursing officer. I admitted that I had become disorganised with my travel returns and explained how I had short circuited the time-consuming system. The nursing officer entered the 1500 miles as private use on my current form, then reported the incident to the district nursing officer.

I was suspended from duty, and on advice from the transport department, the police were informed, who, thankfully, decided not to institute proceedings. As a result of separate enquiries made by the senior internal auditor of my health authority, I was dismissed. After 12 years unblemished, dedicated service, I faced allegations of misconduct with a question mark over my suitability to remain on the nurses' Register. My career was on the line and my livelihood was at stake, due to stupid mis-calculation and poor book-keeping. **”**

Think points

- What part of the Code is in question here?
- What important lessons are there for all practitioners to learn from this story?
- Discuss the advantages and disadvantages of a nursing role that has a large degree of autonomy in practice.
- Discuss the various ways in which community work can put staff into a vulnerable position.
- Given the evidence against the nurse, can you suggest other factors that may have caused this situation to escalate?
- Evaluate the benefits of learner nurses being allocated to the community for part of their training, and consider the difficulties this involves.
- 'The NHS loses millions of pounds annually through waste, fraud and abuse.' Discuss ways in which misuse of resources and property by staff, patients and visitors contribute to this.
- Do you consider this district nurse guilty of misconduct?

The official decision, and discussion

The introduction to the Code of Professional Conduct states, 'Each registered nurse, midwife and health visitor shall act, at all times, in such a manner as to justify public trust and confidence, to uphold and enhance the good standing and reputation of the profession, to serve the interests of society and above all to safeguard the interests of individual patients and clients.'

This district nurse appeared before the Professional Conduct

Committee on allegations concerning excessive mileage claims for financial gain, which she denied. The key evidence rested on a report by the auditor.

He described how he had selected dates from the nurse's diary, and, referring to the patients' addresses, had traced a route to calculate the distance presumably covered, plus an allowance for lunch mileage. It emerged that he had assumed, without question, that the visits were undertaken in the order written down, but the nursing officer confirmed that patients would be seen according to priority of need, not necessarily in the order shown. The Committee members were surprised that the basis of the auditor's calculations had not been challenged by a nurse manager during the previous health authority hearings.

It became clear that the 1500 mile differential could easily have been travelled in the care of patients, even if not recorded, so these charges were not upheld.

The nurse conceded the charges of failing to comply with the health authority instructions but denied any attempt at fraud for financial gain. It took considerable discussion for the Committee to agree that these last charges amounted to misconduct in the strict sense but were an insignificant reflection on her professional competence, so no action was taken against this nurse.

This is probably an example of an incident which should never have reached the UKCC Professional Conduct Committee and which could have been dealt with locally.

Desperate measures

Preparation for practice may be required to extend beyond the basic training, taking account of personal and professional variables and local environment and policies. It is hazardous to throw any nurse in at the deep end, without providing adequate preliminary preparation or ongoing support.

❝ When I completed my RSCN training and passed the finals I was naturally keen to further my career and make use of my hard-earned qualification, but I was disappointed to find that there were no jobs available locally to give me some essential staffing experience.

After scouring the nursing press, the only post which appealed to me (and which I felt able to tackle) turned out to be in a part of the country totally unknown to me. After the initial thrill of getting the job, I found the prospect of a move away from friends, relatives and familiar territory quite unnerving. Shortly after my 21st birthday I travelled alone to Heathcote Hospital.

My reputation preceded me. I looked pretty impressive on paper, with a string of 'O' levels, two 'A's, exemplary ward reports and shining exam passes from a world famous centre of excellence for paediatric care. The nursing officer at Heathcote said I was an answer to their prayers, as they desperately needed qualified staff to cover the busy children's ward at night.

In my heart of hearts I did not feel ready to take charge, but everyone expected me to be far more able, adaptable and experienced that I really was.

During my three-day induction programme I just about grasped the layout of the hospital, met key people in various departments and was briefly oriented to local policies and procedures. It was totally inadequate preparation for my difficult role.

I had expected a period of 'shadowing' or working alongside a permanent member of staff on day duty, to gain familiarity with their methods and approach in the ward.

Instead, I was hastily rushed onto night duty, with the assurance that 'everyone will be pleased to give you any help you require'. But from the outset, the night sister made it clear that I would be responsible for my own domain. Her visits to the children's ward were to be little more than token calls; she emphasised that she had the rest of the hospital to supervise.

Viewing me as the 'specialist', she was content to let me get on with the job – virtually without questions, and without support – as long as everything ticked over nicely.

I was also expected to supervise learners allocated to the ward. Nurse Baker, a second-year student, was experienced with adults but understandably nervous about handling our tiny, unpredictable patients.

My one ally was a highly competent and efficient mature auxiliary nurse. She took on an enormous amount of the routine ward work and helped parents who stayed to care for their children.

Dr Lewis, the paediatric houseman, was also quick to recognise the benefits of my specialist training and, without question, presumed I possessed a high degree of capability and expertise. The more I was able to do, the more he demanded of me.

It was true that during my training I had been exposed to rare conditions and involved with complicated techniques not commonplace for most nurses. At my training hospital it was routine for nurses to prepare and give drug additives to established IVI lines, within the locally agreed procedure.

On Monday, Dr Lewis responded to my call for the top-up due for baby Tang's IVI regime. I had gathered all the equipment ready in a tray for immediate checking and use. The doctor rushed in on his way to the maternity unit, where a baby was about to be delivered by an emergency Caesarian section. He picked up the vial and bag, confirmed that both were correct and returned them to the tray, implying that I would be preparing the infusion.

When I hesitated and reminded him that I was not covered in this district to give IVI additives, he challenged this as nonsense, and said he was sure I had done it plenty of times before. I suppose I should have held my ground and refused, but I was finding it necessary to make allowances in this busy provincial hospital where specialist skills were stretched. Besides, I was due to attend a course soon for extended training, to get a local IVI certificate.

So I asked Nurse Baker to double check each step of the procedure while I signed and dated the infusion chart and nursing notes.

By Wednesday the ward was full to capacity and held a number of very sick children requiring close attention. The situation was made worse by three infants who needed barrier nursing.

In the late evening, nonresident mothers searched for a few words of comfort before leaving their sleeping babies in our care for the night. I tried my best to reassure them and sometimes they broke down in tears as a reaction to the strain of worrying about their sick children.

I had not been used to dealing so closely with these strong emotions and was finding this a considerable burden. I was coming to terms with a strenuous and exacting role, physically, emotionally and professionally, although I was sure that my 'hands on' care of children was unquestionably good.

Close to midnight, Nurse Baker called me urgently to see little Clare, a baby with a chest infection, who was having difficulty breathing and was getting increasingly distressed. I took one look at the snuffly, cyanosed child, with its heaving abdomen, and feared she would suffocate if I did not act fast to clear her nasal passages.

I could see at a glance that there was no piped suction at hand, which I had always been used to, so I decided it would be quicker to rush Clare to the clinic room, to use the Roberts pump stationed with the emergency equipment. But Murphy's law dictated that the machine was not working!

Clare appeared to be getting worse, so I took her to our special side ward, where, thankfully, the portable suction was operating. Unfortunately I couldn't pass the fine suction catheter and guessed that the baby had congested nasal passages. The most effective solution to this would be decongestant nose drops, which I had commonly seen used for infants. Although Clare had not been prescribed Otrivine, I administered two drops to each nostril, believing this was necessary to save the deteriorating baby.

I decided it would be pointless to waste valuable time involving the night sister, so I instructed Nurse Baker to call the duty paediatric doctor, while I continued to try suction on the distressed child. In my anxiety and panic the delay in his response was unbearable. I knew there was only one sure way to get the expert help that this baby urgently required and told Nurse Baker to put out a crash call to summon the cardiac arrest team.

By the time they arrived, my attempt at suction had been successful and Clare was much improved. The paediatric house-man wrote a prescription for Otrivine nose drops, although I did not disclose that I had previously given them on my own initiative. However, there seemed no point in repeating the dose, which could have harmed the child, so I simply signed the prescription chart as given.

In the early morning, baby Clare had the subsequent doses as prescribed and I was relieved that she had made a successful recovery by the time I left duty at 8 am. This had been a most traumatic night, yet ultimately all was well, as my small patient was safe.

I was therefore bewildered to become the subject of an official investigation into my professional performance for giving the un-prescribed nose drops, signing for a dose not given and also giving IV additives without the authorisation of a local extended training certificate. Nurse Baker had, in conversation with a senior member of staff, mentioned the two incidents and questioned their validity.

I was summarily dismissed from my post and, while waiting for the hearing, I started a course on social work at a college near to my home, funding it from occasional auxiliary jobs.

I acknowledged my actions and had indeed signed for them, genuinely believing the baby would die and that I had acted acted in her best interests within my sphere of responsibility. **99**

The official decision, and discussion

Part 4 of the Code of Professional Conduct states that, 'Each registered nurse, midwife and health visitor is accountable for his or her practice and, in the exercise of professional accountability shall acknowledge any limitations of competence and refuse in such cases to accept delegated functions without first having received instruction in regard to those functions and having been assessed as competent.'

Part 1 of the Code states that, 'Each registered nurse [etc] shall act always in such a way as to promote and safeguard the well being and interests of patients/clients.'

The Committee was extremely concerned that this newly registered nurse, who had moved to a job in unfamiliar surroundings, was not given a comprehensive and thorough introduction to prepare her for her role.

Equally reprehensible was the fact that more senior staff led her to believe that she was the expert and there was no point in consulting the 'nonspecialist'. Management appeared to be expecting her to demonstrate the same degree of knowledge and competence, skill and maturity as a practitioner of several years' standing on the Register.

The nurse did not dispute the facts and felt she had learnt a great deal from the unfortunate incident. Although she vehemently hoped she would not lose her right to practise, this nurse had, in the interim, made good use of her time pursuing a new career, gaining excellent references from her college tutors and employers where she did occasional auxiliary work. It is not common for nurses in this situation to make such positive moves and the Committee voiced its respect for these exceptional efforts.

The nurse's actions were recognised as misconduct but, as the Committee felt this nurse was a victim of circumstances, a few words of caution and counsel were deemed sufficient and she retained her registration.

A pawn in the game

A disturbing number of allegations of professional misconduct involve enrolled nurses who have been misused and abused in their role – only to be criticised when they fail to satisfy those unreasonable expectations. It is obvious that many enrolled nurses are treated like pawns moved around the chessboard of service, often utilised dangerously in imprecise, contingency management – amounting to exploitation of the second level practitioner.

> For the most part, I was extremely happy working with the team in the elderly medical unit, but I wasn't always sure of my position. Nor, it appears, was anyone else certain.

As an enrolled nurse, everyone said how useful I was, so flexible and adaptable that I made an invaluable contribution to the ward. How true! When the ward was blessed with students, they were assigned all the 'interesting' cases and I was the dogsbody relegated to the washing and feeding of slow eaters.

When the staff nurse was off, I'd be 'promoted' to complete the routine paper work and check the stores, even required to show the learners what to do. It was assumed I could deal with telephone inquiries and go on the doctors' rounds in Sister's absence. Of course, I'd managed to 'pick up' what to do, because I'd been expected to act up whenever I happened to be the most senior nurse on duty.

On other occasions I was treated like a subordinate and given the duties of an auxiliary. The patients and their relatives found it difficult to comprehend that I could be in charge one evening, and not the next.

Most of my colleagues from our pupil training group reported similar experiences of elevation and demotion in the team hierarchy, slotting into any appropriately vacant space on the duty sheet. We came to accept this as a facet of our value in the nursing service. It produced a muddled service, patchy delivery of care and left staff feeling insecure.

Most of us would have preferred to have clarified our role and were keen to undertake conversion courses. After all, we had to perform a similar role to that of a registered nurse if it suited the service.

My big chance came in Freeman Ward when the second sister left, shortly after our staff nurse had begun maternity leave. As the next most senior nurse available, I was required to work opposite Sister Andrews, and this seemed an ideal opportunity to prove my ability and potential. I enjoyed the responsibility and was encouraged when the nursing officer praised my efforts in keeping the

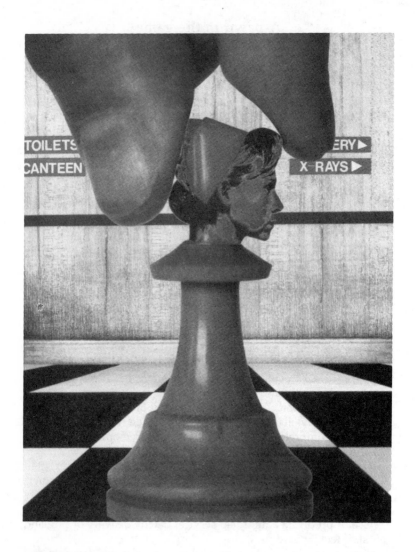

service going during difficult circumstances. She did point out the limitations of my role, but in practice this merely meant having controlled drugs and IV blood checked by a registered nurse.

However, being unfamiliar with the routine of drug administration, I was a bit confounded by the prescription charts and documentation. In one spurt of organisational efficiency, I marked up the index of the CDA record book but, unfortunately, started a new page by mistake. As a result two registered nurses gave a patient heroin only two hours after the last dose.

Originally, I was reprimanded for causing this error in drug administration. Yet, on closer examination of the documents, although the nursing Kardex dictated four-hourly dosage, the actual prescription chart stated a prn. dose within a one to nine-hourly period.

The nursing officer spoke to me after this incident and warned me about overstepping my role, reminding me about my enrolled nurse status. It is difficult to run the ward effectively, while having your hands tied over petty, practical issues.

I continued working well with Sister Andrews, who was delighted to have a conscientious nurse as her partner. But one morning I gave Mrs Taylor her usual dose of heparin, only to be told she was no longer due to have this. I could see nothing to indicate the change, for the badly written prescription entry had not been crossed through, nor was the drug discontinued by signature. It had simply exceeded its valid number of days for administration, but I was accused of acting wrongly.

The nursing officer said that, in the light of this and the previous incident, she was concerned over my performance and felt I was an unsafe practitioner. I tried to point out the defective prescription entry, but I still received a formal written warning. I was suspended for four weeks and allowed to administer drugs only under the supervision of a registered nurse. At the end of that suspension period, I would be assessed by a senior member of the nursing staff to check my competence before being allowed to start again.

In normal circumstances there would be a registered nurse at hand but, although the management expected Sister to supervise me, she was rarely available as she worked on the opposite shift. During my suspension, I was often in charge of the ward and left holding the drug cupboard keys. Yet at the same time I had to call an RGN to supervise and participate in the drug rounds. This could take a long time since most of our patients were old and slow and required considerable help to take their medication. Then just four days before my suspension was due to end, disaster struck.

Sunday mornings are notoriously short staffed and stretched in all of the wards in the geriatric unit. I was in charge of Freeman Ward, working with a student, an auxiliary and an agency enrolled nurse who needed guidance.

I checked the unit duty sheet and rang upstairs to find out if Sister would be available to supervise our drug round. She sounded rather irritated, not unreasonably I suppose, since her own ward was busy and she was preparing to conduct a student assessment. She promised to be down in 10 minutes, expecting everything in readiness.

On our ward round we checked and signed, ensuring that each patient had the correct drugs at the right time. But Mr Holloway needed to make an urgent trip to the toilet just as we were dispensing his pills so, although his chart had been completed, the medicine pot remained with us on the trolley.

Next came Mr Martin who, because he had a sore mouth, needed his tablets to be crushed and mixed with water so that he could take the medicine through a straw.

Not wishing to delay Sister any longer than necessary, I swiftly cleared the trolley and locked the drugs away. All had been completed to her satisfaction. It was, after all, embarrassing, continually having to ask staff to leave their own duties to help me.

As I was clearing up in the clinic room, Mr Holloway popped his head around the door, apologised for upsetting the routine and reminded me that he'd come for his pills.

Oh damn it! His pill pot had been scooped up with all of the dirty ones and I recognised his two tablets dissolving in the soapy washing up bowl. I would not dream of calling Sister again. I also knew this would be a very inconvenient time for the duty nursing officer.

I felt sure that the student and I could check out Mr Holloway's two routine drugs simply, quickly and without fuss. So we did. The diligent student then noticed that the chart was signed and completed, indicating that the patient had already taken his medication.

As a direct result I faced several charges of misconduct relating to this event: failure in not having another member of staff witness the disposal of some tablets; failure to report the untoward occurrence that a patient may not have received his prescribed drugs; failure in instructing a student colleague to check medication even though signed documentation denoted this had already been given.

After this harrowing affair, I was dismissed from my job. Ironically, though, I had no difficulty getting employment **99** elsewhere in the district as a nursing assistant.

Think points

- Which parts of the Code are under question here?
- What might this nurse have done to control the chain of events which conspired to damage her career?
- Discuss the variety of ways in which enrolled nurses, staff nurses and auxiliaries are abused in their roles.
- Discuss the advantages and disadvantages of limiting nurse training to a single grade of qualification.
- State the ways in which nurses may gain professional updating/ in-service training, through their employing authority and through self education.
- Do you consider this nurse could be accused of professional misconduct?

The official decision, and discussion

Part 4 of the Code of Professional Conduct states that, 'Each registered nurse, midwife and health visitor is accountable for his or her practice, and, in the exercise of professional accountability shall acknowledge any limitations of competence and refuse in such cases to accept delegated functions without first having received instruction in regard to those functions and having been assessed as competent.'

Part 3 of the Code states that, 'Each registered nurse [etc] shall take every reasonable opportunity to maintain and improve professional knowledge and competence.'

This case is a prime example of the way in which enrolled nurses are often misused by their managers.

It was considered quite extraordinary that this EN could be suspended from administering medicines for one month, have this 'suspension' confirmed in a letter explaining her to be an 'unsafe practitioner', and yet subsequently be left in charge on 20 shifts.

The Committee was concerned that no relevant training was given during that period to help her to improve her knowledge and competence in the area of drug administration that had been the source of complaint. Nor was there any clearly defined procedure for the proposed assessment of competence following the suspension period. Indeed, three witnesses gave three different versions of the form it would take.

Furthermore, Committee members were profoundly disturbed to discover from the related documentary evidence of the earlier incidents for which she had been counselled and warned, that it had been unreasonable to attach blame to her alone.

One referred to a prescription that was appallingly written and difficult to interpret, while on the other, a medical prescription had been converted into different terms in the nursing notes by nurses more senior than the defendant.

Similarly, in the final incident, doubt had to be cast on the degree of genuine supervision given by the visiting sister. In this instance the EN had been reluctant to call her back, yet was concerned that the patient should not be deprived of his medication.

This enrolled nurse was found guilty of professional misconduct but the Committee agreed that circumstances mitigated the significance of that misconduct. No action was taken against her but the Committee insisted on a public reading of the Statutory Instrument relating to enrolled nurse training. This states the EN's competencies, and thus implies the role for which an enrolled nurse is equipped.

It was obvious that the hospital management had expected the defendant to fulfil a role which far exceeded that for which enrolled nurse training is intended to prepare an individual.

Cruelty and neglect

It is vital that registered practitioners maintain good quality of care, update themselves on professional information and educate others in their caring role. 'Burnout' in professional practice may affect the practitioner who fails to uphold the expected standards required in the varying aspects of her work.

&& In common with many other keen young learner nurses, we expected our forthcoming geriatric module to be less exciting and glamorous than the previous medical and surgical allocations.

But, after a truly inspiring week in block with an earnest tutor, we were pleasantly surprised to have our perceptions altered. She managed to emphasise the encouraging and rewarding aspects of caring for the elderly.

Jenny, Sarah and I were delighted to be working together on a mixed, longstay ward for elderly people. It concentrated on continuing care, with some terminal care and some rehabilitation, which offered great potential for learning.

We were enthusiastic about making the best use of this allocation, enjoying the slow pace of 'low tech' nursing and appreciating the needs of older patients. Here was an opportunity to get to know patients well and develop our skills in formulating care plans.

Unfortunately, from the outset we got the impression that Sister Adams had little concern for her patients as individuals, nor any interest in us as learners.

Naturally, she welcomed our arrival but only as the next 'pair of hands' to help with the daily workload. Any teaching had to be gained from working at the job or from our visiting clinical teacher.

Sister's day was a struggle from beginning to end – ensuring that her 'old dears were fed, watered and kept decent'. It was laborious and demanding work, with few staff, but Sister was obsessed with economy of time. This took precedence over any consideration of individual needs, often to the point of infringing personal dignity and respect.

Nursing notes were a sham. Sister or her deputy, a grumpy senior enrolled nurse, completed them towards the end of each shift, without referring to other nurses. It was conveyor belt care – we were allocated rounds of task-orientated routines, and told, 'It's quicker that way'.

Sister avoided patient allocation, so we never got to know individuals' specific requirements, nor were we able to develop any close rapport. There was little or no planned aim for their care, apart from attending to basic needs and getting them safely through each day.

Many of the old ladies were incontinent because of lack of supervision to take them to the toilet regularly. Even as junior nurses we understood this to be a fundamental approach for the confused or disabled elderly, to avoid the discomfort and shame of incontinence. Consequently, catheterisation was abused and ordered at a whim.

Faecal soiling was equally a problem; no one took the trouble to record bowel action or attend to constipation and overflow. Staff simply moaned at the messes to be cleared up.

Lucy Cranford, who was crippled with arthritis, made the effort, using her walking frame, to struggle from the day area to the toilet. On one occasion she failed to get there in time and understandably had an accident. She stood, embarrassed and bewildered, as the faeces soiled her legs and clothes.

Jenny and I rushed to help and, having cleared the residue, placed a pad and spoken kindly to Lucy, started walking her to the bathroom. Sister was just returning from coffee break and instructed us to wash Lucy down there and then in the corridor.

We hesitated, pointing out that she would be in full view of the staff and patients, both male and female. But Sister said it would be quicker and easier. She sent me to get some equipment while she swiftly undressed Lucy, who stood shivering and clutching onto her walking frame as she was ungraciously cleaned up.

Male patients shuffled in and out and the morning drinks trolley clattered past. I could tell by her expression that Lucy felt utterly degraded and hurt, but she whispered her thanks to us for trying. Unfortunately this type of behaviour appeared to be nothing out of the ordinary.

One Sunday morning I found Miss Utting crying in bed and refusing to get up. Something had obviously upset her, and she was reluctant to speak. I gently encouraged her to tell me what was wrong. It transpired that the night nurse had been angry with her for calling for a bedpan and disturbing the nurse's 3.00 am tea break.

Miss Utting had been addressed curtly, handled onto the pan roughly, and deliberately left on it for half an hour, which had aggravated her longstanding back pain.

We summoned up the courage to report this incident to Sister Adams. She told us not to be concerned and assured us that her night staff were exceptionally good, although terribly overworked.

She added that we were too junior to understand, had never experienced night work and that we should not take too much notice of the patients, because they liked nothing better than to moan about the staff.

Sarah had once seen an auxiliary taunting one of the old men, and enjoying seeing him get confused and agitated. Sister had walked past and must have witnessed this incident, but she said nothing. Likewise, the domestic staff did just as they pleased and were never admonished for pushing patients out of their way or removing unfinished meals when 'time was up'.

Sister rarely stuck to district policy or procedures; she was a law unto herself. She would dispense the pills in the treatment room alone, using her homemade list, saying she knew by now all the drugs her patients were on. Then, taking the tray, she would leave the pots by the patients' beds and somehow expect the nurses to ensure the drugs were administered.

We pupils were getting disturbed and angry about all this and were sure that someone should speak up on behalf of the ward's vulnerable patients. I could not help thinking how dreadful I would feel if my own granny received this sort of care.

Even to our untrained eyes it was obvious that Sister Adams, a qualified nurse on a ward designated as a training area, failed to give any guidance. Her formal instruction was nonexistent and her teaching by example was a liability.

One final incident confirmed our resolve to speak out. Joe was terminally ill and nursed in a side ward. He was floating in and out of consciousness but it was obvious that his life was drawing to a close. Jenny and I prepared the trolley to bathe him and give full nursing care before his relatives arrived.

Sister questioned us as we wheeled the trolley past the office towards Joe's room. 'Don't bother with a full bath, he'll probably die soon, then we would have to bath him all over again,' she said. 'Just tidy him up, do the tasks that are absolutely essential, and be quick about it, there are lots of other patients to attend to.'

Jenny and I were completely dumbfounded and we could not believe we had heard correctly. Being so new, we weren't sure how to go about making a complaint but thought we would have an ally in the clinical teacher.

When we spoke to her she looked embarrassed, as if a can of worms had been opened. She tried to weaken our allegations, although not very convincingly. She muttered about Sister being very experienced, having spent more than a decade in the unit, and made excuses about the difficulties of finding and keeping enough good staff.

Finally, she acknowledged that things were not perfect on the ward, but she felt that nothing could be done to improve conditions and we should leave the matter there. We would be moving on in a fortnight to a different allocation, so it was not really our problem, she said.

But what about the poor patients who were at the mercy of such disgraceful care? Judging from our conversations with other nurses, complaints had been made about Sister Adams before; rumour had it that she had been reprimanded but no appreciable change was seen.

We kept silent until we had left the ward, then we reported our observations to the tutor who had shown such a sensitive interest in the nursing care of the elderly.

She took us to the service manager to repeat these allegations, which led to an investigation, district disciplinary proceedings and a Professional Conduct Committee hearing at the UKCC. **"**

Think points

- Which parts of the Code are under question here?
- Discuss the factors that contribute to burnout in nursing.
- Describe the ways in which burnout manifests itself in personal be-haviour and in professional performance.
- How might the nurse manager have helped this sister to improve her work situation and avoid this blatant deterioration in standards of care?
- Discuss the advantages and disadvantages of having nurse learners allocated to a ward.
- Using your judgement, do you consider this sister should be accused of professional misconduct?

The official decision, and discussion

Part 1 of the Code of Professional Conduct states that, 'Each registered nurse, midwife and health visitor is accountable for his or her practice and, in the exercise of professional account-ability, shall act always in such a way as to promote and safeguard the well being and interests of patients/clients.'

Part 12 of the Code states that, 'Each registered nurse [etc] shall, in the context of the individual's own knowledge, experience and sphere of authority, assist peers and subordinates to de-velop professional competence in accordance with their needs.'

The evidence submitted by the pupil nurses, a report from the director of nursing services about the ward and the sister's job description, were enough to substantiate most of the allega-tions.

Background information illustrated how this sister had been under stress and barely coping with her job for a considerable time. Although these problems had been aired and acknow-ledged, she had not responded to counselling or attempts to help.

It was lamentable to realise that what the pupils had described had probably become an established pattern of personal and professional behaviour. The sister had consistently failed the patients in her care and the learners assigned to her ward for practical supervision.

The Committee was impressed that first year pupils had shown the courage, integrity and persistence to pursue a cause for the rights of patients and the profession, despite encountering difficulties put in their way.

The Committee considered the allegations of misconduct by this experienced ward sister proven. She was removed from the Register and lost the right to practise.

Misplaced loyalties

To illustrate the other side of an allegation about professional misconduct, this story follows the courageous action of one nurse who witnessed bad practice and followed her conscience for the benefit of the patients and good standing of the profession. Unfortunately, she became the victim of derision and abuse for pursuing a just cause.

❝ My life has been thrown into turmoil since I drew attention to a nurse's abominable behaviour in the medical ward. But I insist on following my conscience, which tells me that her actions were wrong, personally and professionally. Yet the treatment I have received for 'stirring up a hornet's nest' could easily have forced me to drop my complaints.

I have become most unpopular, have been victimised and intimidated, verbally abused by some and actively ignored by others. My working life is no longer as enjoyable and contented for I am berated for my 'idealistic' stance and being 'new to the system'. Had I still been a student nurse, I would have worried about the effect on my ward reports but now, as a qualified nurse, I feel an even greater responsibility to challenge bad practice that reflects on the whole profession. A further worry is that my future references could be marred by this incident – the irony being that I was not the one at fault.

While on my last student allocation in the medical ward, I had noticed the tight group formed by the senior, permanent members of staff, who had all worked in the unit for more than 10 years. This hard core, comprising the enrolled nurse, sister and senior nurse, always had the same off duty, always had coffee together, discussed patient care and managed to exclude all other staff. The rest of us knew our place in the 'out group'.

Rita, the enrolled nurse, was a particularly peculiar character; she appeared to have a grudge against the world and took it out on staff and the patients. She was antagonistic to students, making us think that she felt envious and aggrieved at having to stay as an EN.

She was very disrespectful to anyone who was not a white Anglo Saxon Protestant and was fond of referring to people as micks, spades, pakis, jungle bunnies and dib-dobs (Hindus). Yet Rita was humoured and tolerated as a valued member of the staff and a buddy of Sister – no one seemed unduly perturbed that she muttered these offensive jibes under her breath.

We had a devout Catholic patient in the side ward for investigations, being visited by his wife. The couple had requested that the priest come to give a blessing of the Sacrament of the sick and asked for preparations to be made for his visit. Back in the clinic room,

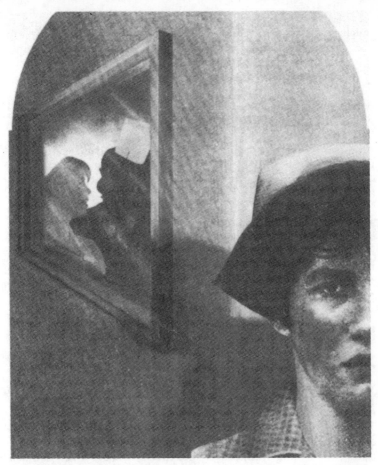

Rita sneered at their need for 'smells and bells' and their 'holy regalia', then chuckled like the bigot she was.

I was horrified and could see by her shy, embarrassed look that the wife had heard the remark. I learned later that she complained to Sister, who had promised to reprimand Rita.

As a student I got on with my ward work as best I could, although this was hardly a good learning situation. In my senior role, close to finals, I tried to influence the atmosphere as much as possible and the learners helped one another care for the patients.

Rita had little patience and was always moaning that we were mollycoddling the old men, whereas she would think nothing of slapping patients to urge them on. One chap with Huntington's chorea had such poor co-ordination that he could not fend for himself or follow instructions. Rita would pull this man around roughly and once flung him bodily into an armchair, causing the poor man to cry out.

A colleague and I witnessed this and other assaults and, after much deliberation, decided to complain to Sister. She listened to our story and promised she would investigate. Happy that something would be done, I left the ward and concentrated on my final examinations which, thankfully, I passed.

Some weeks later I overheard a student talking about Rita, whose behaviour had not altered one iota. We compared experiences and I wondered why nothing had been done about her misdemeanours.

I wrote to the sister to inquire about my complaint. A reply came from the senior nurse who told me the matter had been investigated and dealt with locally. I considered this unsatisfactory because I had never been called to make a statement with regard to any investigation.

I tried to elicit some details of the case by writing courteously to ask about the investigation, since I, as the complainant, had not been called to give my side of the story. It was suggested that I make an appointment if I wished to discuss the matter further. I met the senior nurse and the senior manager, who still gave no answers to my specific questions. It was implied, and pressure was put to bear, that I should accept that the complaint had been satisfactorily investigated and resolved. I was thanked for my conscientious observations but there was a strong suggestion that I should let the matter rest.

I realised that I was facing an impossible task, for these three people were defending one another in a web of collusion that no outsider could penetrate. I was incensed by this rotten situation where patient care suffered in the midst of corruption and poor nursing was permitted to exist, thanks to a cover-up.

I was distressed at this state of affairs and knew that other nurses agreed with me and could corroborate my evidence. They urged me to take my complaint directly to the UKCC, which I finally did in a long, detailed letter, concerning the original incidents, the failures to pursue complaints and subsequent concealment.

I also sent a copy of my letter to the director of nursing services, who immediately initiated an investigation in the hospital. At this stage, two undated documents miraculously appeared in the enrolled nurse's folder, to indicate that an investigation had been made and a report filed.

During the year waiting for the UKCC hearing, positive action was at last taken locally to unravel the tangle of deceit.

It appeared that the sister could not believe the allegation of Rita's unkind behaviour, as she had known her for so long. The sister was sent on a development programme, which enabled her to recognise her initial failure in her handling of the incidents; it would also assist her in future action on complaints procedure.

Similarly, the senior nurse had been misguided and influenced to accept willingly the sister's conclusion. She had failed to make her own inquiry and had seriously transgressed her managerial role. Here was a nurse thrown into a senior role, without adequate preparation or support, who has since benefited from in-service management training and was demonstrating a renewed interest in her post.

The enrolled nurse was normally a caring and tolerant person, who, it was recognised, had become institutionalised and unmotivated after working in the same ward for a number of years. Following a refresher course and allocation to another ward, where her performance was carefully monitored, Rita was reported to be making a great impression and was given excellent references.

Meanwhile, my original charges stood with the UKCC, and it was a year of living nightmare for me. I suffered a terrible loss of face, which made it difficult for me to continue working in the hospital, but I was determined to stick it out.

Staff were divided. Some felt I was right to publicise the intolerable state of affairs. Many said they wished they had the guts to do as I had done but feared the backlash of hostility, some of which I was experiencing.

Others called me a 'scab', a 'grass', a 'tell-tale', a 'disloyal goody-goody', and said I would make everyone nervous if they felt they were being 'spied on' at work. Mine appeared to be the greater sin to report the wrong doer and *I* was made out to be the guilty one. It strikes me that many people have misguided loyalties, if they put protection of bad staff before upholding the profession and good care. **99**

Think points

- Which parts of the Code are under question here?
- Discuss the degrees of misconduct and reasons why a nurse may choose to report a colleague to the professional body.
- Discuss the reasons why a nurse may be reluctant to expose a colleague who shows poor professional behaviour.
- In your area of work, can you pinpoint situations where you witnessed malpractice or abuse of patients, how you felt and what action you took – or did not take.
- Discuss what may motivate a nurse to make false accusations against a colleague.
- Discuss the conflict of upholding professional conduct versus staff loyalty.
- How may a strong group of permanent staff be (a) beneficial and (b) detrimental to the functioning of a ward or department?
- Using your judgement, do you consider these three nurses guilty of professional misconduct?

The official decision, and discussion

Part 6 of the Code of Professional Conduct states that, 'Each registered nurse, midwife and health visitor is accountable for his or her practice, and, in the exercise of professional accountability shall take account of the customs, values, and spiritual beliefs of patients/clients.'

Part 2 of the Code states that 'Each registered nurse [etc] shall ensure that no action or omission on his/her part or within his/her sphere of influence is detrimental to the condition or safety of patients/clients.'

During the days before the UKCC hearing, student and newly qualified nurses verified the evidence of abuse by the enrolled nurse. The Catholic couple were brought as witnesses to corroborate the derogatory sectarian remark – and that no action was taken by the sister on the original complaint.

The Committee considered the reprehensible actions by the EN and noted that she had contravened the expectations of practitioners in a number of ways, especially failing to accord respect to customs and spiritual beliefs of the patient. The sister and senior nurse had failed in their managerial roles and had been unduly influenced by friendships.

All were considered guilty of misconduct but due regard was taken of the positive steps made by the DNS to rectify the problems. The nurses were all now performing well and understood their faults, so no further action was taken apart from giving advice.

The Committee praised the new staff nurses and the one in particular who had pursued her complaint to achieve proper investigation in spite of numerous obstructions and intimidation.

It was obvious that this conspiracy of silence and a collusion of staff was broken only by the courageous and persistent actions of these nurses to bring the situation out into the open. They demonstrated immense personal stoicism and an awareness of their professional responsibility as stated in the UKCC Code of Professional Conduct.

It is a salutary reminder that it is also professional misconduct to turn the other way and fail to report a misdemeanour observed.

Home from home

The Code of Conduct is relevant to all qualified nurses in every sphere of practice, reaching wide to afford protection to the public and ensure standards are maintained within the profession. Independent private nursing homes, without the benefits of any supervisory or controlling management structure, could easily become places of abuse and neglect in the hands of unscrupulous nurses who renage on their responsibilities.

      I am Nigel Taylor, Managing Director of the Gemini Group of Nursing Homes for the Elderly. We are developing our services here in Seacroft, which attracts a lot of retired people. It is inevitable that many of those people will require skilled nursing care as they get older, more frail, lose their faculties and their independence.

When the company was looking at investment business options, our advisers had recognised the potential in the nursing home market for an increasing elderly population. We were recommended to get established in Seacroft, which seemed ripe for expansion.

There are obvious benefits in having a large organisation running a group of nursing homes, thereby centralising stores and catering, having managers to arrange the accounts and to undertake various administrative duties. Nevertheless, we are bound by the regulations of the health authority, are subject to their inspections and depend on our registered nurses to uphold the standards of care in each home.

I had guessed there were some ailing owner-occupied homes in Seacroft that we might usefully acquire, saving us having to make the structural alterations needed to convert private houses. My hunch was rewarded when I placed a magazine advertisement and received a number of interesting replies.

Elizabeth Monkton was keen to sell her property as a going concern and had been looking for a buyer. I certainly liked the sound of Meadow View, set in spacious, attractive grounds, within 200 yards of the sea. Miss Monkton, acting as matron and proprietor, had built up her home as a respectable viable business over the past six years, and it was always fully occupied with 30 paying residents.

My company had engaged the services of a nurse adviser, experienced in managing nursing homes, so she accompanied me on the initial visit.

Miss Monkton was most welcoming and took us on an extensive tour of the home. The fabric of the building was in good repair and the interior decor was pleasing. The fire escape and fireproofed doors met with regulations, as did the storage of medicines and facilities for food.

113

While I discussed the financial side of the business with the proprietor over coffee, the nurse adviser made a more detailed examination of individual rooms, talked with some residents and found out about their daily agenda. She agreed that, although the standard of care was satisfactory, there was plenty of scope for improving the day-to-day management.

Having finally decided that Gemini Nursing Homes would like to buy the property, we employed Mrs Jan Elliot, RGN, to be the prospective matron of Meadow View.

With the legal paperwork completed, it was arranged that Gemini would take over the business within two months. Mrs Elliot arranged to interview the existing staff at the home, with the exception of Miss Monkton, who was planning to move up to Scotland to live with her sister.

It was unfortunate, but Mrs Elliot found the staff unsatisfactory. She was unimpressed by their attitude to the elderly people for whom they were caring.

To them it was merely a convenient job; they were a little *clique* of pals and had no intention of altering their ways to suit a new matron. As one of them said, 'Betty has always been pleased with our work; we see no reason for change.'

Mrs Elliot wondered who actually ran the home, for it appeared that Miss Monkton's practical involvement was minimal. Our matron finally decided to employ just one person from the present team, Sara, a bright young nursing assistant who appeared to welcome the infusion of new management and progressive ideas of care.

Recruitment of the necessary replacement staff was soon completed and Mrs Elliot was ready to start with a fresh team at the home, from deputy matron, nurses and domestic staff.

Everyone was excited and enthusiastic when the day came to finalise the change of ownership at Meadow View. As arranged, I joined Mrs Elliot, the deputy matron and the rest of the team to take over the home at 8 am on a cold January morning.

We were horrified by what we found. On entering the home, we noticed immediately that the place was filthy and we were struck by an overwhelming stench of urine and faeces.

Naturally, we searched to find out who was in charge, so they could explain this scandalous state of affairs, but the only staff member present was the assistant, Sara, the sole survivor of the transition. She was struggling to look after the residents but it was impossible for her to make even the barest impact on the care that was required for 30 highly dependent, elderly people scattered in individual rooms.

None of the residents had been given breakfast nor was there any evidence that preparations were under way. On further inspection, there were no provisions available for substantial meals.

Full praise must be given to our new team who, spurred on by anger and compassionate concern, set to work cleaning up the residents and offering them warm nourishment. Without exception, everyone knuckled down to relieve the distress.

Mrs Elliot and I explored the premises, taking full account of the lamentable scene which I, as a lay person, found shocking and nauseating. Every resident was dirty and unkempt. Many of these elderly people had dried faeces covering much of their body, which suggested it must have been there for some time.

The rooms and bed linen were in a dreadful state. Underneath many of the beds there were large quantities of foul linen and excreta-laden, soiled incontinence pads, which had obviously just been thrown there and left to accumulate over a number of days.

Our last, heart-rending find was in a small, unheated room, which, according to the plans of the home, was used as a temporary mortuary for the deceased awaiting collection by the undertakers. In this chilled room, on a cold winter's day, we discovered a very frail old lady, who looked emaciated and obviously ill, and who was profoundly dirty and neglected.

The whole deplorable situation was difficult to comprehend. We finally found Miss Monkton in her flat at the top of the building where she was casually packing in readiness for her departure.

She gave no explanation for the state of the residents and was quite unperturbed by our remonstrations and complaints. She simply said that it was now our premises and everything was our responsibility. This ex-matron continued folding her clothes into her suitcase, giving us hardly a glance of acknowledgement.

Sara was able to shed some light on recent events. Several staff had left soon after they knew they would not be re-employed by the new management, feeling the urgent need to get similar jobs in the area. Others had waited to receive their large pay packet – reflecting Christmas overtime – then had left, without any replacement staff being recruited to take over. Miss Monkton had remained resident to provide nominal registered nurse cover but there had been a severe shortage of staff for several days and a lack of essential supplies.

I followed Mrs Elliot's recommendation that we ask the inspecting officers of the health authority to visit immediately to ensure independent corroboration of the state of affairs at the point of transfer of ownership.

The inspectors arrived within two hours and, although many of the residents were cleaned up and the worst contamination removed, they were able to see for themselves and record the terrible condition of the residents and the home. They had last made a planned visit for formal inspection four months previously and agreed that standards had now deteriorated to a totally unacceptable degree.

We checked with the inspectors about our rights in this instance and were advised that a complaint could be brought against the outgoing matron/proprietor. Charges brought before the Professional Conduct Committee of the UKCC were to the effect that Miss Monkton was guilty of having neglected old and vulnerable patients and had failed to provide a **99** suitable environment for their care.

Think points

- Do you consider the ex-matron in this case to be guilty of professional misconduct?
- If so, what decision would you consider appropriate? Would you:
  (a) Postpone judgement for a stated period and set criteria for a resumed hearing when the option of removal will remain available?
  (b) Remove the respondent's name from the Register with immediate effect?
  (c) Leave her name on the Register but administer words of caution and counsel?
- Are there any other lessons to be learned from this scenario?

The official decision, and discussion

Following its standard procedure, the UKCC served a formal notice of the hearing to Miss Monkton. However, she neither attended in person, nor sent anyone to represent her in her absence. Furthermore, there was no written evidence in her support.

As Miss Monkton had been self-employed for a number of years, both at Meadow View and at previous owner-run homes, it was not possible to supply the Committee with details of her history. Several witnesses were called to describe the circumstances relating to the charge and the Committee was satisfied that these were proven and constituted professional misconduct.

Without the opportunity to question Miss Monkton and form an assessment of her character and her view of the situation, the Committee felt it had no option but to remove her name from the Register with immediate effect.

The Committee expressed concern about the inspection of nursing homes in Seacroft and drew these concerns to the attention of the registering authority. Notably, there were insufficient staff available for the inspection of the rapidly growing number of nursing homes in this area. In particular, inspections were less frequent than desirable and were always conducted when advance notice had been given of an impending visit.

Action not prescribed

When duty takes client care outside of the familiar and protective hospital setting, nurses encounter new dimensions of responsibility. Accountability means taking decisions and being able to justify them. Nurses acting on their own authority must be certain that their actions are for the ultimate benefit of the patient, for decisions will be judged within the full context of the situation.

❝ April was a month of busy preparation for the holiday in which I was to accompany eight people with a mental handicap to a hotel in Sandford. I had been surprised when our unit manager made the initial suggestion, because more senior nurses had not been offered the opportunity. She had said, however, that in my two years as a staff nurse I had shown myself to be competent, conscientious and resourceful. In short, she had confidence in my ability to do the job well.

The holiday sounded a little daunting at first, but it was also a new experience which promised to be pleasurable and would help my professional development. I took it as a compliment that my senior managers considered me fit to take on this responsibility.

The group of residents selected were not from the ward I worked in but from adjacent Jay Ward. I made it my business to visit Jay several times to get acquainted with the residents, to find out about their capabilities, degree of independence and medication, and, equally important, for them to get to know me.

Roger Finn, the assistant nurse from Jay, who would be the only other staff member on the trip, knew the residents well. After several evenings discussing the holiday, finding out about entertainments and planning excursions, Roger and I felt that a good week lay ahead. We were determined to make this a holiday to remember for the clients, none of whom had been further than the local village.

Sister Robinson gave me a thorough verbal and written handover and discussed each prescription to ensure I was familiar with it.

Roger and I helped the holidaymakers with the last of their packing, while Sister prepared the metal drug box, which was then locked and the keys handed to me.

We loaded our belongings into the hospital minibus on loan for the trip. Roger and I had been cadging things for the holiday, so in went cricket bats and stumps, a football, swingball, foldaway chairs, picnic baskets, some board games and a pack of cards.

With Roger and seven men in the back it was a tight squeeze but Tommy Davis revelled in the view from the front seat next to me, the sole driver. Before long the singsong started and, once they got underway on *10 Green Bottles*, the group was in fine voice.

Our hotel was most comfortable and the staff couldn't have been more helpful. Being used to handicapped visitors, they were understanding and had the right attitude, so we soon felt at home.

Naturally, part of the purpose of the holiday was to encourage correct social behaviour, so it was important to ensure that our residents kept their rooms tidy, washed and dressed appropriately and observed table manners in the dining room. We were surprised how well they responded to the hotel atmosphere and how much they enjoyed being waited on at the table.

After our day out at a local zoo Tommy was so excited that he had difficulty sleeping and his constant chatter disturbed his room mate. When I checked, his chart carried a prescription for Mogadon at night, as required, but there was none in the medicine box. Nor, I discovered, were there any of the other drugs 'as required'.

Roger found this surprising because, although Tommy did not often need night sedation, it did become necessary at times when he became overexcited. Roger could not understand why Sister Robinson had not taken the precaution of including some medication for him. As we did not want a repeat of the previous night's sleeplessness, I considered how best to get the drugs. It would be pointless to contact the hospital, a long distance away, when our need was imminent.

Trevor, another resident, was getting alarmed about his constipation, brought on by the change of diet, and was asking for some of the yellow liquid to 'make him go'. I decided the best option was to seek help from a local GP, who was most supportive in the circumstances and issued relevant prescriptions. He found it a little strange that we had come so far and were not prepared for such eventualities – but so did I.

Our holiday was blessed with beautiful weather, which enabled us to enjoy plenty of outdoor activities – cricket on the beach, crazy golf, and even a spot of paddling. It was an action-packed week, full of new experiences which seemed to have a beneficial effect on all the residents; it was really most rewarding.

There was a noticeable improvement in several men; they had often shown noisy, aggressive and antisocial traits but now behaved well. Roger commented on the calm and co-operation, the animation and interest produced by this change of environment and group involvement.

Having witnessed this change for the better in behaviour, I decided to omit the lunchtime dose of Largactil for three of the men, as it seemed counterproductive to suppress their activities in the middle of the day. I did not seek authority from the hospital but made a professional decision based on my knowledge and training, and I was constantly observing for any adverse responses. Consequently, the residents were more alert and able to join in all the fun.

We had a wonderful week and were sorry when it came to the end. Roger and I helped the men pack their belongings, making them check under the beds and in the bathroom. I packed the medicine box, including the prescription sheets, and locked it securely.

After saying our final thanks and farewells to the hotel staff, we took the men on one last trip to the amusement arcade to use up their remaining pocket money. The return journey was memorable because of the delays through heavy Saturday traffic and work sites along the route, in addition to a couple of refreshment and toilet stops.

We arrived back at Jay Ward at nine o'clock in the evening, feeling exhausted. I officially handed over responsibility of the residents to Sister Robinson, together with the medicine box and keys. I explained that, although I was now on annual leave, I would return on Monday to complete my report and clear up any remaining details.

On Monday morning I met Trevor outside Jay Ward and stopped for a chat. Sister Robinson greeted me sternly at the entrance and indicated that I should wait in the doctor's interview room while she contacted the senior nurse manager. I was bemused by her tone and her actions.

When the senior nurse manager arrived I was told I would not be allowed into Jay Ward, nor into my own ward, because I was suspended from duty on full pay, while an investigation was conducted into discrepancies in the contents of the medicine box.

I was given no opportunity to explain the circumstances, nor was I asked for information. I was sent home to wait for an investigation by the hospital managers.

At a local disciplinary hearing I was dismissed from employment and referred to the UKCC Committee of Professional Conduct.

It was alleged that I behaved improperly by obtaining prescriptions from a GP rather than calling the hospital, and that I withheld prescribed medicines from residents. **„**

Think points

- As a member of the Professional Conduct Committee, would you consider that these allegations amount to misconduct in a professional sense?
- What might this story teach us about accountability in nursing? Accountability for the grassroots nurse? Accountability for nurse managers?
- Take this opportunity to familiarise yourself with the two UKCC advisory papers on *Exercising Accountability* and *Administration of Medicines*.

The official decision, and discussion

This staff nurse had been regarded by his managers as capable of bearing the burden of responsibility for the care of residents on holiday and had been invested with that authority.

The medicine box had been assembled inadequately by a more senior nurse, who had better knowledge of the residents. She failed to include the 'as required' drugs, even though records demonstrated that these were occasionally needed. The staff nurse had sought the most effective solution in the circumstances to remedy the omissions.

The staff nurse admitted that he withheld some behaviour-modifying medicines, which resulted in discrepancies in the medicine box. However, he attempted to justify his actions and persuade the Committee that his good intentions did not constitute misconduct.

As the only specialist nurse present, his decision was based on sound professional judgement from observing improvements in behaviour and was taken in the interests of the residents in his charge.

The members were astounded that this case had come as far as the UKCC Professional Conduct Committee. Far from acting in a manner which could be regarded as contrary to the interests of the residents, this nurse had respected and served those interests by his willingness and ability to exercise professional judgement. He understood clearly that he was accountable for that judgement and was able to defend this before a committee of his peers.

It appeared that this nurse was being criticised for his willingness to exercise personal judgement in unusual and demanding circumstances and for adopting a more flexible approach than was normally practised.

The matters which had occurred were not regarded as professional misconduct by the Committee and the case was closed.

One big headache

Violence and aggressive outbursts can be expected occurrences within any psychiatric setting. Nurses trained to care for the mentally ill must recognise potentially explosive situations and use their skills to defuse them.

They must be careful not to fall into the trap of 'winding patients up', in the teasing style of the old custodian, who shows no respect for the psychiatric patient as an individual with real needs and feelings. When hostilities arouse emotions, it is difficult to determine whether any ensuing violent reaction is self defence or a blatant attack.

❝❝ Kent Ward was apt to have a volatile atmosphere, and skirmishes were not uncommon. This mixed acute admission ward, in a psychiatric unit of a district general hospital serving a large area, had a busy turnover of acutely ill and often disturbed patients.

Because aggression is not uncommon in psychiatric hospitals, nurses can sometimes regard it as an occupational hazard. During our training we examine the factors which may contribute to disharmony and anger: features of certain illnesses, stimuli in the environment, clashes with other patients or staff, and frustration.

We also learn how best to deal with aggressive outbursts in safe, non-judgemental ways. Those clear cut, well formulated policies on the management of violence look impressive on paper and represent the ideal. However, it is a different matter always to act appropriately and correctly, to conduct oneself 'by the book', when caught up in the urgency and immediacy of a spontaneous affray.

But, by anyone's standards, what I witnessed one Friday afternoon defies interpretation as rational, professional behaviour.

I was working with the late-shift team, led by Charlie Harris. He was an experienced charge nurse, who had been on Kent for a number of years. But, although still a young man, he was rather stuck in his ways. Charlie was a conscientious nurse but rather a plodder, reluctant to get involved with new ideas, not bothered about progress in the ward or advancing in his own career.

Charlie was returning from days off, so needed to be acquainted with the news, especially about our two new patients. The handover covered all the essential points, but seemed rather hurried – the morning staff gave the impression they were anxious to get away for the weekend.

There were obvious priorities: three patients recovering from ECT, a suicidal girl needing close observation and a disoriented man in the habit of wandering off.

Brian had been newly admitted in a severe anxiety state and was to be seen by the psychologist. Gloria Thomas, in her early fifties,

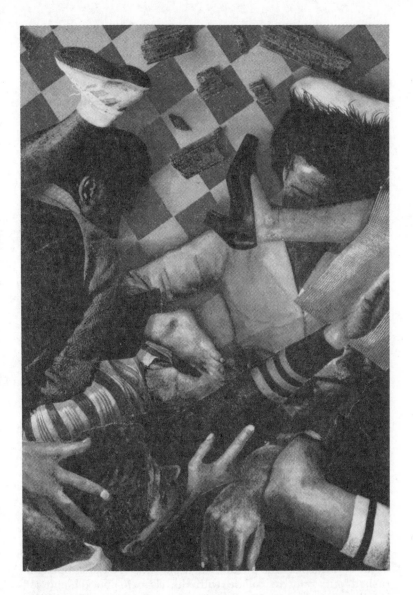

was the other admission, complaining of depression and showing marked agitation. Charlie remembered Gloria vaguely from a previous admission and tried to find out more about her condition. He asked if there was an invalid husband at home, recalling something to that effect from earlier days.

The doctor was to come up later to see Gloria, who was dismissed as 'attention seeking', as she had a tendency to follow us around.

Sister slung her bag over her shoulder and fumbled in her pocket for the drug keys, tossing them to Charlie. He and I made a start on the afternoon medicines; patients collected their drugs around two o'clock, and a queue was already forming.

I went inside the clinic room to double check the medicines, as Charlie dispensed them from the trolley which barred the doorway. We were coaxing Martin to take his elixir and the others were getting a bit impatient. Gloria barged into the front of the queue and, looking flushed and angry, demanded something to treat her headache, since she had been waiting all morning.

Charlie knew nothing had been prescribed, but said he would arrange for this when the doctor came. 'Hell, what do you have to do to get some service around here?' Gloria shouted as she walked away. 'All they do is fob you off. No one takes a blind bit of notice. I only want a lousy aspirin, not the crown jewels!' Her voice echoed down the corridor.

As we completed the drug administration, Charlie handed me the medicine pots to wash. Gloria had returned to the clinic room in a most determined way, obviously exasperated, and stood in the doorway with her clenched hands on her hips.

'Look, sunshine, I've had enough, do you hear, enough! My head is splitting, give me something,' she yelled at Charlie.

He remained unmoved, repeated his previous statement and turned to tidy away the medicine bottles. I thought that his coolness and intransigence, as well as his silent exercise of power, could be provocative to someone already angry.

Gloria shouted at him, 'I've been asking all bloody morning and not one of you offers any help. Call yourselves nurses? Just rubbish, all of you. Why doesn't anybody listen?'

Charlie replied casually, 'It's the first I've heard of it.'

Suddenly, Gloria lunged forward and thrust her hand towards the medicine containers. But Charlie slammed the lid of the trolley down, catching Gloria's arm and hand, causing her to cry out. This added to her fury and, with a string of abusive words directed at Charlie, she raised her arms as if to hit him.

From behind, I saw Charlie take a heavy swipe and land a punch on Gloria's jaw. She fell back reeling and ended up flat on her back in the corridor. Charlie pushed the trolley into the clinic room and rushed out, only to collide with the cleaner's bucket and fall headlong beside the patient. He managed to get up and called me to help move Gloria.

She put up a struggle as we carried her, with some difficulty, to the small dormitory close by. Charlie nodded towards the nearest bed and it appeared a simple proposition to place Gloria on it. Unfortunately, the bed wheels were not locked. As we lent our weight against the bed, it rolled away and the three of us collapsed in a heap on the floor. Gloria continued to resist, swearing loudly and liberally as she battled to get free.

Martin appeared in the dormitory and, with the kind of wit sometimes seen in the hyperactive, asked if we were teaching Gloria judo. Without waiting for an answer, he entered into the spirit of things, picked up a chair and gave us all a hefty whack.

Other patients who had come to investigate the commotion also joined in the action, until the floor was littered with a tangle of fighting people. The ward staff rallied to our rescue but it was necessary to call other nurses and the unit manager before order was completely restored.

It did not sound plausible when we came to explain how this situation had escalated out of all proportion. Starting with a dissatisfied, disgruntled patient seeking relief from a headache, there had developed, within a few minutes, something resembling a riot in the ward.

Investigations followed relating to the incident and, in particular, about alleged ill-treatment by the charge nurse.

Think points

- Would you agree this action constituted misconduct?
- Can you suggest ways in which Charlie might have handled this situation better at the outset?
- What valuable lessons might the student have learned from witnessing and participating in this event?
- What stereotyped ideas about people admitted with a psychiatric illness appear to be supported in this story?

The official decision, and discussion

Charlie admitted that he struck Gloria but argued this was in self defence. Evidence from witnesses, the student nurse, the domestic assistant and Gloria herself, corroborated that the charge nurse had intentionally punched the patient on the jaw. This is the standard of proof that the law requires, so the Committee found the allegation proven and agreed that it constituted professional misconduct.

Judging this action in context, it was noted that the morning shift staff had given an inadequate handover report, leaving Charlie with insufficient information about the patient. There was no mention that Gloria had been complaining of a headache and had been asking for pain relief during most of that shift, nor what action had been proposed – if any.

The ward was adequately staffed at the time of this incident. Charlie's manager stated that he had been a satisfactory employee, although there was concern that he was reluctant to accept change, took no initiative and lacked imagination.

The Committee expressed concern about the limited attention given to the patient and her requirements by the morning shift and of their incomplete handover. However, this did not justify or excuse the charge nurse's actions in response to her request.

It was decided to remove this nurse's name from the Register. A transcript of the hearing was sent to the chairman of the health authority, in order to draw his attention to matters of concern about the management of the unit.

When the crunch comes

Practitioners must ensure that their actions remain within the parameters dictated by their professional role. To take on other duties and to fail to adhere to correct policies and procedures leaves a nurse professionally vulnerable.

Nurses must stand their ground, understand their limitations and their accountability, and never be persuaded into unauthorised activities.

❝ After 10 years of intensive care nursing, there was not much that I had not seen or dealt with, and I was considered an expert. I had taken a job as senior sister of the intensive care unit at Rocksley Hospital nearly four years before, so I could live closer to my parents.

The unit was smaller than in my previous hospital, but it was well staffed, with reliable permanent nurses who pulled together as a team. I settled quickly and enjoyed the close-knit, co-operative atmosphere that is so necessary in a stressful, high-tech environment. We were familiar with ventilators, central venous pressure lines, intravenous infusions and caring for highly dependent patients balanced between life and death.

Our ICU provided an interesting variety of work, as we were taking in patients from all over the hospital. We were used to a rapid turnover and lurching from crisis to crisis. Patients were admitted from the accident and emergency department following accident, collapse or overdose. Patients also came directly from theatre following complications during surgery. We received cardiac patients, and those transferred directly from general wards.

There was something invigorating about working in ICU, something special about the thrill and excitement of critical care nursing. Nurses had to develop the stamina and resilience to cope with urgent daily problems, responding with speed and accuracy.

Our expertise was recognised by the doctors who admitted patients to our unit. Frankly, it was difficult trying to remember which patient belonged to which doctor, who might be held up in theatre, or in an outpatient clinic or on pressing business in his general ward. Junior doctors changed posts with such frequency that the qualified nurses on ICU often knew more than these youngsters straight from medical school.

It was a nightmare trying to contact one of them quickly when a crisis occurred. We were lucky that Dr Francome was usually available; she was the consultant anaesthetist with authority for the overall medical administrative control of the unit.

Margaret Francome would do a morning and evening round to check each patient. She had great confidence in the nurses, many of whom she had worked with closely for a number of years. We could always anticipate her needs, because we were familiar with her approach.

If Margaret was occupied on a long case in theatre, we could not disturb her and we would only summon the crash team in event of a dire emergency. Margaret always made sure that patients were prescribed analgesia and sedatives which might prove necessary in her absence.

It was also an unwritten rule that, if a cardiac patient had persistent bradycardia with accompanying hypotension, any one of the registered nurses was authorised to administer a routine dose of atropine to get him stabilised without delay.

Sunday afternoon was not the best time to develop heart problems, but Mrs Timmins luckily got the last bed in the intensive care unit. She was admitted from A&E by the medical team. The senior house officer rang through with her details, explained that she had an infusion set up, was on a monitor, and that he would be in later to check her condition.

Mrs Timmins was very anxious and obviously shocked. Although relieved to be admitted to ICU, she was worried that this carried serious implications.

Student Nurse James was allocated to admit Mrs Timmins and I asked her to stay with the patient to provide some comfort and reassurance. After completing the forms, Nurse James was recording Mrs Timmins' vital signs. The patient's temperature was (not unexpectedly) a little raised, but her pulse was getting slower and her blood pressure was low.

I checked the observations myself, watched the monitor, checked the readings again and conferred with the staff nurse. Unfortunately, this was Dr Francome's weekend off and we had to rely on the duty anaesthetist, who, I knew, was busy in theatre, or the assigning team, who were occupied in A&E.

The staff nurse and I decided the criteria matched those indicated by Dr Francome, which would justify the course of action we had taken on many similar occasions. I gave Mrs Timmins the atropine, which would speed up her heart rate and raise her blood pressure. The staff nurse and I carefully checked the drug and signed the drug card to that effect.

I asked Nurse James to stay with the patient and monitor the readings at quarter-hourly intervals, while trying her best to allow Mrs Timmins to get some rest. Our routine work continued for the other patients and the nurses took tea breaks in relays.

An hour and a half later the two medical team doctors managed to visit their patient. By this time Mrs Timmins' observations were looking more healthy and the doctors told her they were pleased with her progress.

At that moment Mrs Timmins burst into tears and got quite hysterical. 'You can tell me, doctor, don't hide the truth. I'm going to die, aren't I?' she said.

Dr Hesketh, the registrar, looked dumbfounded and asked why she would think that. 'My brain is going,' she said. 'I feel strange, I can't see you properly. That's a sign, isn't it? And my mouth is so dry.' The poor woman sounded increasingly distressed and despairing.

'Oh, that's the effect of the atropine,' I explained. 'Don't worry, that will soon wear off.' Dr Hesketh asked his senior house officer why atropine had been prescribed, but he looked equally bewildered.

Nurse James settled Mrs Timmins, while the staff nurse and I escorted the doctors to the nurses' station. I explained that I had given the drug, after checking the criteria with my registered nurse colleague, and on an understanding with the head of the unit.

Dr Hesketh was extremely displeased with my interference, despite the fact that no harm had come to the patient. He asked to see the prescription authorised by Dr Francome, but there was nothing actually prescribed in writing. It was simply a verbal agreement between Dr Francome and the nurses working in ICU.

The staff nurse said that this was our regular practice and that we all understood the necessary criteria. It was a recognised way of speeding up care to patients in urgent need of standardised treatment.

The registrar thought this was a slack way to run an ICU and an action fraught with danger. Suppose something had gone wrong – who would be prepared to take the responsibility? He did not approve of other people meddling with his line of treatment and said that nurses had no right to decide on prescribing.

The staff nurse and I told him that we had the authority and support of our senior medical colleague, naïvely believing that this would protect us.

Dr Hesketh brought the matter to the attention of the district nursing officer and I was sacked, pending an inquiry.

I do not know if Dr Hesketh ever confronted Margaret Francome, but she did not give written evidence to the Investigating Committee of the ENB. Nor did she appear as a witness when my case was subsequently heard before the Professional Conduct Committee of the UKCC. Presumably she had been advised, as doctors usually are, not to jeopardise her own **99** career in support of a nurse.

129

The official decision, and discussion

When the detailed circumstances were heard, this sister denied that she had given an unprescribed drug, and nursing colleagues supported her evidence concerning the verbal authorisation. Dr Francome never appeared to corroborate or deny her role in the incident.

The Professional Conduct Committee decided the facts were established – that a drug was given which had not been prescribed properly. The Committee members were not prepared to accept that a general, undocumented instruction could be regarded as a prescription. Ultimately the case rested on the professional accountability of the sister. Her action was judged as misconduct in the professional sense. Before the Committee decided on a course of action it heard further information at the mitigation/aggravation stage.

The nurse manager provided an excellent testimonial, confirming that, until this event, the respondent had been a highly satisfactory ICU senior sister. It was unfortunate that an earlier, similar incident in her former job had remained on record at the UKCC and was revealed at this stage. Five years earlier, in the ICU of another hospital, she had been found guilty of giving unprescribed drugs, once again convinced that she was doing the best for patients.

On that occasion, the Professional Conduct Committee found misconduct proven but decided to postpone judgement for a year. As she had a sound work record and recommendations from her managers, she was cautioned and given professional advice, but remained on the Register.

From the evidence of this case, and considering the history of this respondent, the Committee decided to remove the nurse's name from the professional Register.

Buried under paper

Maintaining updated records is an important and necessary aspect of work for every professional practitioner. It is all too easy to consider this a tiresome burden and a waste of valuable time that could be better spent on client care. Practitioners must resist the temptation to fall behind with their paperwork, as this could challenge professional performance and prove a costly failing.

66 There are times when I think I shall be snowed under by the amount of paperwork required in this health authority. I cannot believe that the duplication and repetition of information improves the care of clients – quite the opposite. Can't managers see that my valuable time would be better spent on practical tasks than on futile form filling?

When I joined this health centre three years ago, I could see great potential and, at interview, my prospective colleagues appeared to welcome my proposals. It was easy to see why. The place was pretty chaotic, needing organisation and a splash of initiative to renew motivation and co-operation.

There was considerable bickering and interdisciplinary tension, resulting in many staff changes, which caused disruption and disharmony. I started sensitivity group meetings to air and share our ideas and grumbles. I also introduced sessions on communication skills and counselling, which everyone enjoyed and found beneficial and refreshing.

I felt it important that I should 'stretch' myself personally and professionally, in addition to the considerable amount of routine work, which involved running antenatal classes, parentcraft sessions, health education clinic and GP work, alongside my allotted caseload of nearly 400 children.

In addition to my regular work with new families and the under-fives, I set up a postnatal support group. This was especially helpful in giving confidence and companionship to mothers who were adjusting to having a first baby. As a single parent myself, I could understand many of the difficulties these women might experience and I believed it important to develop this aspect of my health visitor role.

In our practice, details of every under-five client were kept in a birth book, which had columns for each examination and test result. I carried this with me on visits and to clinics and was meticulous and methodical at keeping these individual, personalised records up to date.

Health visitors were required to duplicate much of this information by completing separate cards to itemise each of the large

131

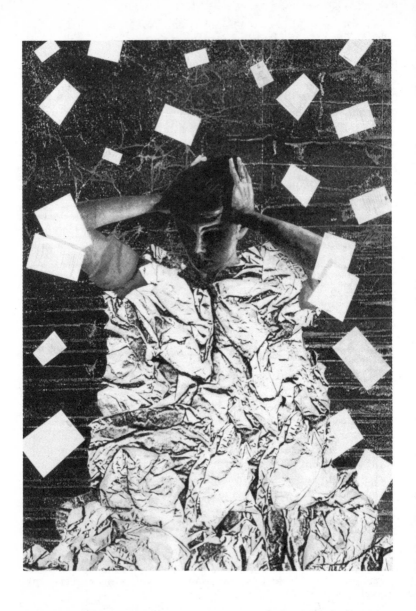

number of tasks performed. It was decidedly laborious, took up much precious time and I wondered how necessary and useful this repetition was. Hearing tests, periodic developmental screening, phenylketonuria test results and immunisation checks all had to be documented, along with other details already recorded in my birth book.

Some of the information was used for liaison with other departments; we had to forward immunisation consent forms to the appropriate clinic, for example. There was also specific notification to the community physician, and data sheets to be sent to the pre-school health section at the appropriate time.

Other information seemed to be more of an administrative nature – maintaining a diary, recording all visits, trips and lectures given, mileage claim forms, monthly returns on our workload to the nursing officer and so on. I think anyone would agree that we were enveloped in an inordinate amount of paperwork.

I was not consciously refusing to maintain those 'secondary' records, but it was one of those jobs that could be shelved, especially when more pressing problems required attention.

The part time secretary, originally employed to assist with the health visitors' amassed clerical work, had long since been 'misappropriated' to do a variety of other office jobs in the health centre. Although I had asked my nursing officer several times to help resolve the clerical situation, she offered no assistance and implied that if I was experiencing difficulties, I might not be up to my job.

So it happened that some cards were consigned to my drawer to await that quiet moment that somehow never materialised. On those odd occasions when I felt a twinge on guilt, I was reassured by the thought that each child's personal file was correct and up to date, readily available for quick reference.

Nevertheless, I was aware of my deficiency with documentation, and on my self assessment appraisal form, registered this as one of my shortcomings. In an open and honest appraisal meeting with my director of nursing services, I admitted that this was my Achilles heel. I explained how I had asked my nursing officer to chase me up for the monthly returns she required to improve my performance.

Meanwhile, it was gratifying that my influence was having a powerful and positive effect on staff working relationships at the centre. A colleague and I were proposing a new joint project to give specialised support and guidance to a group of teenage mothers, which seemed a neglected area of care.

Our nursing officer was trying to rationalise the caseloads of the four health visitors, as the disparity between our work levels required some reallocation. She had requested a count of our clients and other responsibilities, which I had not managed to complete before going on holiday.

During my absence, the nursing officer had access to my files and discovered a number of discrepancies in my record-keeping. Together with a colleague, she carried out a thorough investigation, which revealed considerable problems related to my paperwork, including non-completion of primary record cards of children for several months or years, no entries regarding hearing tests or PKU test results, immunisation consent forms and preschool data sheets not forwarded to the relevant sections, and gaps in my diary entries in respect of mileage claims and visits.

I was unable to explain the situation to my nurse manager, nor did I understand the enormity of this failure. Despite the many positive aspects of my work, I was sacked and called to appear before the Professional Conduct Committee of the UKCC to answer charges of misconduct regarding **99** omissions in my records.

Think points

- Do you regard this practice as misconduct and, if proven, what recommendation would you make for this health visitor's professional future?
- Can you think of times in your area of work when you are confronted with 'excessive documentation'? How do you feel about it and how do you cope with these demands?
- Can you suggest ways in which this health visitor might have better managed her difficulties relating to record-keeping?
- In the context of this story and other nursing situations, discuss how excellence in some aspects of a role does not excuse laxity in other aspects.

The official decision, and discussion

This experienced health visitor appeared unrepresented before the UKCC Professional Conduct Committee to defend a total of 15 charges alleging misconduct concerning official documentation.

The nursing officer described how discrepancies contravened local policies, although she failed to mention the birth book record until challenged by the health visitor. The defendant correctly pointed out that she had impeccably maintained this record pertaining to all children, as required by the health authority, which should also be checked by nurse managers. She demonstrated a detailed knowledge of families in her care which could only have resulted from frequent visits and a great interest in her clients.

It was revealed that the health visitor had requested to see the DNS with the critical self appraisal that had exposed earlier difficulties with record-keeping. Formal appraisal of staff by their managers was not being conducted annually as intended.

Nor did the nursing officer consider it necessary to monitor her health visitor practitioners unless a specific query or complaint needed pursuing.

In her mitigation, the health visitor described a number of impressive innovations featuring in her practice, and many testimonials were submitted in her support. Previous employers sketched a picture of her exemplary career, high standards of care and concern, together with her leadership qualities.

While she accepted responsibility for her failures and admitted the facts, the defendant felt the reaction to them had been excessive in relation to the rest of her performance.

The Committee agreed that the facts constituted professional misconduct. However, they noted that she was an enthusiastic, innovative and committed health visitor, with good personal and professional qualities, caught in a climate of change and disagreement. In acknowledging her own shortcomings in record-keeping, she had recognised an issue that needed to be addressed personally.

This practitioner required guidance from a manager who would ensure that she attended to the basic necessary tasks before embarking on new ventures, while still encouraging innovation.

The Committee decided to take no further action on the proven misconduct, so this respondent retained her registration and was able to resume health visiting practice.

As a result of this case, the health authority made substantial changes in its system of monitoring, management, appraisal and induction of health visitors.

The Chairman of the Professional Conduct Committee reiterated that maintaining adequate records was both a fundamental feature of practice and professional accountability. Clause 2 of the Professional Code of Conduct makes an omission to do something for which you have responsibility just as serious as an act of commission.

Taking unfair advantage

The public hold nurses in high esteem and rely upon professional integrity to ensure there are no corrupt practices. However, within the privileged caring relationship, opportunities always exist for dishonest nurses to take advantage of their clients.

By gaining the trust and confidence of clients, the nurse has a tremendous amount of practical and emotional hold over people who depend upon her care and, ironically, require the greatest protection. It is not difficult for the determined nurse to violate her professional position for personal gain.

66 The financial realities of home ownership made their impact when the bills began pouring in. After struggling to raise a mortgage for my modest terraced house, other unforeseen expenses appeared, as I tried to make my new home modern and comfortable. It was getting increasingly difficult to match these debts with my salary as a district nurse.

My district nursing practice, in a rural area, with a reasonable caseload, allowed me adequate time with each of my clients. Many were elderly, housebound and living in some isolation, so they invariably welcomed a visit. Clients would enjoy a chat over a cup of tea, for some barely saw another living soul during the rest of the week. Naturally, I was able to build up good relationships with the people in my care and, before long, they trusted me and took me into their confidence.

Mrs Williams had a kindly neighbour who collected her pension every week and delivered essential groceries, together with the even more essential cigarettes. Her remaining cash was accumulated in the house. I came across a packet of £5 notes between her clean towels in the airing cupboard and suggested it would be safer in the bank.

'Don't trust 'em, never 'ad no use for 'em, not gonna start now at my time of life,' was her curt reply.

What if she should get robbed? I asked, trying to make her see the folly of her ways. But she said the money was distributed in secret places, in dribs and drabs all around the house; thieves would never find it. Some was in the Toby jug, some under the cutlery drawer and, in a very unoriginal hiding place, some more was stitched into the mattress!

What if there should be a fire? I said; she would lose everything. But no, Mrs Williams had told her son there was £1000 secure in a tea-caddy, buried in the garden by the lilac tree, to pay for her funeral. What more did she need?

This lady was convinced that her money should be around her for safe keeping and no persuasion on my part could change her mind. I wondered if she remembered all the hiding places or knew exactly how much she had altogether. She got confused at times during bouts of chronic bronchitis.

In the course of my visits I discovered that a number of elderly clients held the same opinion about banks, and it appeared commonplace for them to retain substantial amounts of cash on their property.

I could not erase the thought from my mind. Here were old people, comfortably off in homes that they owned, with no plans for structural alterations or refurnishing, gathering money for which they had no real need. While they were sitting on a nest-egg, I was sitting on a financial time bomb, which could devastate me and for which I could see no solution.

Mrs Williams was thrilled to learn that a bed had been reserved for her at the general hospital for surgery to correct her bunions. She was hoping that, once her feet had been fixed, she would be sufficiently mobile to take a slow walk to the local shops on fine days, and when her chest was trouble-free.

As her son was on holiday, I volunteered to help Mrs Williams pack, before the hospital car came. She was most grateful, knowing it was my day off, but I dismissed her thanks, saying it would only take half an hour. The old lady said that I was a jolly good friend to her.

Mrs Williams sorted some reading material, while I got her a selection of clean clothing and washing items. In nearly every cupboard and drawer I found hidden packets of folded money. I am ashamed to say that the temptation was simply too great and I helped myself to some cash. A couple of fivers from under the towels, a few more from the underclothes drawer, some stray notes from the bathroom cabinet and others from a vase. I was convinced she would never notice they had gone and I doubt she had any idea how much she actually possessed.

When Mrs Williams was packed and ready to go, the car arrived, but she insisted on a final check around the house. Meanwhile I wrote a letter to the ward staff, in my capacity as the district nurse. I described Mrs Williams' health and social status, mentioning that she was an ardent smoker and apt to get confused when she had chest problems. Everything I said was true and I felt the hospital might appreciate a warning about her anaesthetic risk or reaction, but I also wanted to cover my tracks in case she complained of money being missing.

I was £200 richer, which eased my debt with the bank. The simple and foolproof execution of the theft encouraged me to act again. After all, who would listen to an old person with a history of confusion? Indeed, who could ever prove what money had been on her premises in scattered notes?

In Miss Babington's case things were even more straightforward. She was being transferred to sheltered accommodation, because her senile dementia made it impossible for her to manage alone at home. There would be no question that she was confused, disoriented and might even demonstrate some paranoid ideas that people were 'after her money'.

Once again, I detailed all this information in the letter to the home warden, after I had helped to pack Miss Babington's belongings – and helped myself to cash in her cottage.

By now, understanding the 'problem' of old people keeping money in the house, I made it my business to discuss their financial affairs in the hope that they would make better arrangements. During our talks, they usually told me the safe hiding places they used. Sometimes I just happened upon money during the course of my work, which required opening drawers.

Two clients were due for a month's break of respite care in the local cottage hospital. The staff there knew me well, so they had no reason to doubt either the excellent nursing care given to my clients or details of their fluctuating mental state. When these ladies complained of losing money, the staff simply dismissed this as part of the confusion and a natural reaction to a change of environment.

However, a daughter of one lady questioned her mother more closely and discussed the matter with the sister of the ward. The daughter declared that her mother had always been perfectly lucid and queried my transfer comments as a fabrication. She was further alerted to examine her mother's grievance when she learnt that I had volunteered to go in my off duty to help pack 'as a friend' rather than in my official capacity as district nurse.

The daughter pursued her inquiry through my nursing officer, who was astounded by the accusations. Before long the police were involved in charges relating to robbery. I was no match for their thorough investigation and crumbled under the exposure of my mounting debts and large bank deposits, all of which coincided with the transfer of a client.

My case was heard in a criminal court and I was found guilty of thefts totalling over £2000 from six clients I had visited. From being a highly respected district nurse, I was now a common criminal, branded with a conviction. Thankfully the judge was lenient because of my previous unblemished history, service to the community and the undue pressure of debt, so he imposed a suspended prison sentence.

For this second chance I was extremely grateful, and prepared to rebuild my life afresh. However, I found out that when a registered nurse, midwife or health visitor is found guilty in a criminal court this information is always passed to an Investigating Committee of the relevant National Board. If the conviction appears to have bearing on the professional performance of the practitioner, this will become the subject of a professional conduct **99** hearing before a Committee of the UKCC.

Think points

- In your opinion, what are the most disturbing features of this case?
- Do you think this action is worthy of the removal of the nurse's registration?
- Which types of criminal offence reported to the National Boards are most likely to be considered to have a bearing on professional performance? Explain how these could adversely affect a nursing role.

The official decision, and discussion

The facts were established by the certificate of conviction. A Professional Conduct Committee is always bound by the outcome of guilt established in a court of law. It must accept this as conclusive evidence and act on that verdict without further question.

The district nurse had declined to attend the Committee hearing, had chosen not to be represented, nor did she submit any mitigation for consideration.

A nursing officer spoke highly of her former employee, having always considered her to be a skilful and caring district nurse who formed excellent relationships with her clients. This nurse had been well liked, respected and, above all, perhaps ironically, was trusted by the people in her care and their relatives.

The nursing officer was obviously distressed at having to give evidence. She had been shocked that such allegations had been made and subsequently proved against a nurse whom she had believed to be a person of honesty and integrity.

The Committee said that this district nurse had seriously abused her privileged access to the homes and property of an extremely vulnerable, dependent client group. She had clearly contravened several parts of the Code of Conduct and it was agreed that her behaviour constituted professional misconduct.

Members regarded it as particularly nasty and devious that she would step in and out of her professional role, going as a friend to help pack but reverting to the nurse role to write misleading notes about the alleged confused state of clients.

As clients went to different places at different times, this lessened the risk of linking individual complaints that might expose her guilt.

Despite the positive caring and competent qualities in this practitioner's favour, the Committee felt that she should be removed from the Register, in the public interest.

Condoning ill treatment

Within the leadership role, a senior nurse may have occasion to reprimand staff on the team. Regard for the patients' rights and needs must take priority over loyalties or friendships amongst colleagues. It is against the Code of Conduct to turn a blind eye that allows bad practice to go unheeded and unchecked, for the act of omission is equally serious as the act of commission.

66 As a staff nurse on the male psychogeriatric ward, I had been interested to learn of the new policy towards integration. It was considered therapeutic to have men and women mixed together in our wards.

Although I agreed with the idea in principle, I was not so convinced when I heard that our male patients would be transferred to Emily Ward. There were no plans for structural alterations, yet it appeared that men and women would be sharing the same dormitory and toilet facilities.

We protested about the practical difficulties and inadequacy of resources, mentioning also the dignity, modesty and self respect of our elderly patients. Management assured us that it was a necessary and progressive move, but screens were the best solution they could offer. Unfortunately, even these were tatty and in short supply. Only we understood that confused, demented, wandering old folk were no respecters of mobile screens.

Sonia Wilson, the very able senior sister of Emily Ward for the past 12 years, was the natural successor to head the team of the new combined ward, with myself as senior staff nurse.

We worked well together and devised various strategies to ensure that this new project worked to the patients' advantage.

The bathroom would be reserved first thing in the morning for the women, while the non-urgent men could wait until after breakfast. We also decided that some evening shaving would take the rush out of the morning routine.

Two toilets were reserved exclusively for men and two for women, with coloured symbols marked on each of the doors. The most agitated patients would be allocated to the side rooms, so as not to disturb those sleeping in the dormitory.

Mixed activities, such as bingo and quizzes, craftwork and a gentle exercise class, took place in the central lounge. The patients seemed to enjoy the company of the opposite sex, provided they weren't too intrusive. But not all the staff found the move so stimulating, for it had been an upheaval and it added further pressure to their normal duties. However, I was pleased that the male and female teams integrated so well – too well in some instances.

Peter Quinn exuded an old-world charm mingled with humour and frankness. As a nursing assistant he proved a great asset, being a thorough and efficient worker with an obliging and friendly manner. He was a reliable and willing person who became a cornerstone of our team and was always keen to do overtime to help out.

Sonia Wilson and Peter found they had a lot in common, having northern roots and being members of the local drama group. They were often seen chatting together in the social club.

Despite my earlier reservations, the integration was working reasonably well. We had plenty of staff for this pilot scheme and there was good team cohesion, although the physical environment remained far from satisfactory. A shortage of linen and bedclothes was our biggest headache, especially having so many incontinent patients.

Peter was getting noticeably slack, taking unacceptable short cuts in his work that jeopardised the patients' privacy. One Sunday morning, while the vicar was holding a service in the lounge, Peter escorted two male patients through, who were wearing only short pyjama tops. A few of the women giggled, but others looked very embarrassed.

I followed and asked Peter what he was doing, making it clear that this was totally unacceptable behaviour. He argued that it was not his fault that the linen ran out at the weekend and that he was doing his job as best as circumstances would allow.

I disagreed and, knowing that Sister Wilson was in the office, I was disappointed she did not offer her support. It seemed strangely out of character for her. A fortnight later I had cause to reprimand Peter again and we had a fierce argument. After I spotted him carrying Jimmy Hanson stark naked down the ward, in full view of both male and female patients and some astounded relatives, I challenged him.

My remonstrations were loud and strong, audible to anyone in the vicinity – I was somewhat surprised by the extent of my own fury. Yet Sister Wilson, who was checking stores in the clinic room, failed to get involved in our row or question what was happening.

When I tried later to explain what took place, Sister refused to intervene in something that was my province and that I had handled satisfactorily. Maybe she had a point. But within another two months a further incident occurred which seriously questioned her professional practice.

Peter Quinn had patients lined up in the day room for evening shaves and was making great headway. Mr Barratt was agitated for some unknown reason, but Peter insisted on forcing him into the seat by the sink. Two enrolled nurses were tidying the day room when they witnessed an act of incredible callousness.

Peter Quinn lathered up the shaving soap, then deliberately forced the soapy brush into Mr Barratt's mouth, which caused him to splutter and choke.

The ENs immediately shouted at Peter to stop and rushed to assist the poor, distressed patient, who was by now yelling and thrashing about.

On hearing the sudden noise and commotion, Sister Wilson poked her head through the connecting hatch from the kitchen. She took no action and said nothing. Instead she withdrew and continued to prepare the night drinks trolley, muttering that the routine work was already behind schedule.

In the handover report, Sister Wilson had the honesty to warn the night nurses about Mr Barratt's condition.

In a matter-of-fact way she explained that they were not to worry if Mr Barratt began foaming at the lips; he wasn't having a fit, he'd simply had his mouth washed out with soap. She gave no further details, leaving the nurses bewildered by her coolness at the patient's plight.

Sister Wilson's attitude left much to be desired in a qualified nurse. The culmination of these events resulted in a health authority inquiry and her subsequent appearance before the **99** Professional Conduct Committee of the UKCC.

Think points

- Can you suggest reasons why the sister had apparently decided to relinquish her responsibility to correct certain staff members on her team?
- Discuss possible factors within the relationships of these characters that caused friction and tension between the staff.
- Can you suggest ways in which these interpersonal and professional difficulties might have been resolved locally?
- Considering both the long term and recent performance of this sister, would you consider it appropriate that her name be removed from the professional Register?

The official decision, and discussion

During hearings of the Professional Conduct Committee, in respect of evidence, the standard of proof legally required must satisfy each member beyond reasonable doubt that the incidents actually took place.

In the first two incidents cited by the staff nurse, although he believed the sister had observed unacceptable behaviour, there was no definite proof that she had in fact witnessed these. So these two allegations were not upheld and the sister not required to answer charges.

Concerning the shaving soap incident, the facts, corroborated by the enrolled nurses and night nurses, were proven beyond doubt.

Peter Quinn also gave evidence, but naturally, being neither a registered nor an enrolled carer, he would not be subject to any disciplinary procedure by the UKCC. In this context, his behaviour was not being questioned but, instead, the actions and responsibility of the registered nurse to whom he was answerable.

Sister Wilson appeared to have condoned the appalling and inexcusable ill treatment of a vulnerable patient. Her subsequent remarks were considered prejudicial to the welfare of the patient and contrary to proper professional attitudes.

In the mitigation/aggravation stage, there were testimonials from a number of hospital staff and several relatives in support of her exemplary work as a ward sister.

Sister Wilson's employers had found her work most creditworthy over the years, with the exception of the period when Peter Quinn had been allocated to her team. She had been subjected to local discipline and, when transferred, gave a highly satisfactory performance.

The Committee agreed that the charges amounted to misconduct. However, in view of the respondent's exemplary career record both before and after the period under scrutiny, it was decided to postpone judgement. At a resumed hearing one year later the Committee would reconsider the situation, in the light of her performance and references, one of which would be required from a direct-line manager.

The Committee added how appalled it was to find that those responsible for hospital management had rushed the integration of elderly male and female patients without first ensuring that there was appropriate ward design and adequate resources.

Stretched to the limits

If people are stretched beyond capacity, dangers lurk in lost concentration, poor decision making and excessive demands that compromise performance. When mistakes do occur, it is open to interpretation as to who might be held to blame for the poor environment of care. Managers who permit their staff to cope in unsafe and intolerable conditions may find they have more of a case to answer than the individual who finally succumbs to the inevitable mistake.

66 Our nights had never previously coincided but I knew of Sister Woodman by reputation. A good midwife, an excellent teacher, methodical and diligent, but painstakingly slow. Unfortunately, in the busy labour suite we needed people who knew how to 'put their skates on' when pressures demanded.

Before the horrific night under scrutiny I had already sent a letter to our district nursing officer, to alert her to the intolerable pressure of work and low morale in the midwifery unit. I was backed by several colleagues.

We had not had even the courtesy of a reply, so we continued struggling to paper over the cracks. The health authority seemed to have been comforted by a press report that implied staffing was satisfactory. We knew this to be a fallacy and had fears about the inherent dangers.

When I took charge at the 9 pm handover, there were three mothers in established labour, including Mrs Stapleton, in the single room, with a known intrauterine death. Obviously she and her husband would need a great deal of support at this traumatic time.

Mrs Pereira, in delivery room one, had been admitted that morning, in labour with her second child. A cardiotocograph (CTG) was attached to monitor fetal heart rate and movements. The labour was progressing safely and satisfactorily.

A young primipara was in delivery room two. A further four patients in the six-bed ward had been given Prostin pessaries earlier that evening and were resting comfortably.

The two student midwives on duty, both only three months into training, were being supervised by Sister Woodman. I had overall responsibility for the labour suite, together with my individual clinical duties. I allocated patients to staff to ensure continuity of care, while I took charge of Mrs Stapleton.

My tidy arrangements did not last long, however. By 10 pm two more women had been admitted, one of whom appeared to be on the verge of a pre-term labour at 26 weeks. The nursing officer responded to my request for help by sending a staff midwife from

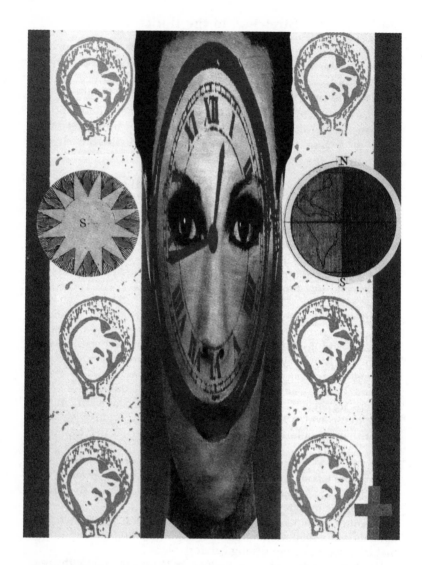

the antenatal ward, boosting coverage to five staff members for nine patients.

An hour later our previous admission did go into pre-term labour and we were faced with anxious parents and the imminent reality of a very premature infant needing specialist care.

I organised meal breaks to begin early, in order to maximise staff cover later, when I anticipated there would be a greater workload. Another midwife came to relieve over this period and admitted yet another woman in labour just after 1 am. For most of this time there were three staff rotating between 10 patients.

At 1.45 am I managed to grab a snack, and soon after returning from my break I noticed that Mrs Pereira had a raised temperature. The doctor on call prescribed an antibiotic. There were no other problems with this patient and her CTG tracings were in order. The nursing officer, who was visiting on her rounds, confirmed the observations.

Although she could see we were frantically busy, she offered neither her personal assistance nor help from elsewhere in the unit. There were five staff, two of whom were in training, to care for 10 patients in various stages of labour, with one pre-term labour and one intrauterine death.

Sister Woodman seemed oblivious to the increasing pressure of activity and refused to take on responsibilities other than her original patients. She was not prepared to absorb any extra duties, complaining bitterly of already being too busy.

By 5 am, it was evident that Mrs Stapleton was due to deliver and would need my undivided attention, so I arranged for one of the student midwives to oversee Mrs Pereira.

Knowing I would be occupied, I urged Sister Woodman to hurry with her work and help the other nurses. She had been involved in a delivery with the other student and was lingering over the post-delivery routine, starting a discussion that could easily have been postponed to a more convenient time. Other mothers were in need of her attention now, but she refused to be hurried and I was frustrated by her attitude.

Within half an hour Mrs Stapleton had delivered the dead baby, a perfect little boy. It was unfortunate in these circumstances that the third stage was complicated by a broken cord and retained placenta, eventually expelled by maternal effort. I had recently attended a study day on stillbirth and was acutely aware of my role at this delicate time. The parents shared their grief and were prepared to accept a photograph by which to remember their son.

When I telephoned the nursing officer to inform her of the dead baby, I asked for assistance from another midwife, as a number of women were nearing the delivery stage. She sent an auxiliary, which was no surprise to me, for this had become routine practice.

Back in Mrs Pereira's room, I quickly noted that the CTG tracing had dropped to 60 on two occasions, but had subsequently returned to 160. If it dropped again, I knew I would need to call the doctor.

I was then summoned to the outside phone, where I confirmed with two consecutive husbands that their labouring wives should be admitted.

By 6.30 am, the suite was at full capacity, with 12 patients and six staff, but only three registered midwives. Sister Woodman continued to busy herself supervising the students. It was obvious that we needed more appropriate staff at this point. I felt exhausted by a variety of emotional and physical demands pulling me in all directions.

By 7 am, I was involved with an imminent delivery, so I asked the staff midwife to check Mrs Pereira, before she admitted one of the new women. She also noted a dip in the CTG but, because of its subsequent revival to a normal reading, it did not give rise to obvious concern.

A student midwife was then left to observe Mrs Pereira, along with several other patients. When the day staff arrived at 7.30 am, I took the midwife into the delivery room to hand over the care of Mrs Pereira.

Only then did I recognise the significance of the fetal heart tracing that had failed to register with me earlier. It contained huge decelerations over a long period of time and now there was meconium liquor on the pad, both indicative of fetal distress. I immediately summoned the obstetric team by crash call but, despite their efforts with an emergency forceps delivery, the baby was stillborn.

My actions became the subject of allegations of misconduct before a UKCC hearing. These were: my failure to take appropriate action when the CTG trace was suggestive of fetal distress, failure to seek medical advice and allowing Mrs Pereira to continue expulsive efforts for too long. The errors were **99** unthinkable for any experienced midwife.

Think points

- Do you consider this midwife's action constitutes misconduct and, if so, should she lose her right to practise?
- Do you believe any other people could be held to blame for contributing to this tragedy and, if so, might you wish to make any recommendations?
- How might you best deal with members of staff who do not pull their weight in the team?

The official decision, and discussion

The solicitor representing this midwife suggested a procedural ploy to ensure that the Committee would be presented with the full evidence in context. So she denied that the facts constituted misconduct, although accepting their essential accuracy. As anticipated, a number of issues caused grave concern to the Committee members.

On that night the workload had been excessive, while the

response by the managers was inadequate, and it appeared that such poor staffing levels were not unusual. This practitioner had already drawn the attention of senior managers to these difficulties, as the Code of Conduct requires.

The nursing officer stated that she did not normally offer assistance unless first receiving a request and her managerial style could best be described as 'non-interventionist'. Sister Woodman emerged as a person inclined to do no more than she absolutely had to and who determined her own pace of work.

Both midwives failed to appreciate the extent of their roles and had a distorted view of their professional accountability.

The director of midwifery services spoke highly of the respondent, as a knowledgeable, competent, motivated and respected practitioner, holding the advanced diploma in midwifery and due to study for the midwives' teachers' diploma.

Many impressive letters of support were submitted by former colleagues. The Stapletons had sent their thanks for her kindness and support, which reflected the amount of time devoted to this couple on that occasion.

In retrospect, the midwife agreed the CTG tracings were obviously disturbing. In normal circumstances she would have responded earlier and appropriately to avert such a tragedy. It was an error in her practice to allow labour to progress and she totally accepted the responsibility. She could only say that, having been so engrossed with her allocation of patients, general pressure of work and supervision of the department, she had failed to absorb and comprehend the readings.

Although the finding of misconduct was proved, no further action was taken against this respondent. The Committee agreed that she could clearly see her error and had learned from this disastrous lesson. However, she was the unfortunate victim in an inadequate environment of care. A transcript of the hearing was sent to the health authority Chairman, with an expression of the Committee's concern over matters emerging from this case.

Talking in confidence

The personal information about clients must receive respectful and confidential handling by nurses. However, the matter of confidentiality is not as straightforward and clear cut as might be expected.

    ❝ I welcomed the chance of an interesting career move when I applied for the post of community psychiatric nurse (CPN). My prospective employers did not seem concerned that I had neither experience of community work nor specific training, although they promised to send me on a CPN course when a vacancy occurred.

Meanwhile, they were satisfied that my RMN qualification and two years as a night charge nurse at an acute psychiatric unit were suitable preparation. As I had been a mature student, and had taken up nursing as a second career in my middle years, they acknowledged that my experience in the 'university of life' would be a considerable bonus to the job.

Talk about being thrown in at the deep end! I was appointed to *establish* a community psychiatric nursing service to cover the district, with immediate responsibility to the director of nursing services for primary care. She was less than enthusiastic about this extra responsibility foisted on her and I felt unable to look to her for support.

With no inpatient psychiatric facilities, my health authority had to rely on services from the neighbouring authority of Snaresborough.

I inherited 50 clients from the CPN who had been providing a visiting service from Snaresborough, but soon my caseload grew out of all proportion. I was disappointed that my role had disintegrated into offering a crisis intervention service, rather than providing the ideal of support and therapeutic care.

Able to demonstrate a need, I persuaded my manager to employ extra staff. Chris, also an unqualified CPN, joined me, and six months later a third nurse made up the team.

Because of an increasing caseload during my time alone, I could not be spared from work, so I missed the opportunity to attend the CPN training course. Instead, I spent two days at a workshop which was an introduction to the role of a CPN.

By the time the next course started I was so disillusioned and frustrated with the community psychiatric service that I had decided to look for a different job. Chris took the course placement and handed over half his clients, who became my responsibility in addition to my own caseload.

One of our clients, Roger Ford, was considered high risk because he had made two serious suicide attempts in the past four months.

On the first occasion he had deliberately crashed his car into a lamp-post and had to be admitted to hospital.

He then took a hefty overdose of a cocktail of drugs, needed a stomach wash-out and was admitted to the general hospital. After the psychiatrist from Snaresborough had seen Roger in the medical ward, he asked me to prepare a social report before making any decision for care.

I did not like to admit that I had never been involved with a social report. Acting on my initiative, I followed the format from a report Chris had prepared on another client, using it as my model.

When I first visited Roger in hospital he was too ill and drowsy to talk much. On my next visit, later in the week, he was better physically but hostile and abusive, resisting all my attempts to offer support or help him deal with his problems.

I was able to determine the cause of much of Roger's anger and the probable reason for attempting to end his life. Intense family and marital difficulties had recently come to a head. His wife Georgina had left him, taking with her their two young children. She had moved into the house of a woman friend with whom she was having a lesbian relationship.

It was important to get her side of the story, so I visited Georgina at her new home. In a very distressed state, she explained that Roger had been threatening her, her partner and the children with violence. They were not empty threats, she believed, and she was genuinely worried, because Roger had several convictions for theft and acts of violence.

Still unsure that I had the full picture, I went to see Peter Harris, head of the engineering department at Snaresborough College. I had been told that he was Roger's friend and employer, having been instrumental in getting Roger a job at the college.

At the outset of our discussion, we confirmed that Peter would be speaking on behalf of Roger, and as a friend. My aim was to clarify whether Georgina's allegations about her husband's convictions and behaviour were true.

Peter confirmed that Roger had initially attended the college on a course for the unemployed. He had done well and shown such natural flair as an instructor that he had been given a job to teach basic engineering skills to unemployed young people. At the time of this interview Roger was in his college post, on leave from the psychiatric hospital.

I told Peter what Georgina Ford had said about her husband's violent threats. When I asked him if he knew whether Roger had a criminal record, he became guarded and agitated. He refused to confirm or deny knowledge of this information.

I explained that I had no way of knowing if the allegations about convictions were true and had no means of checking. I reiterated that I was sharing this information and making inquiries of him only because he was a close friend of Roger's.

Mr Harris told me to go away and put my allegations in writing, otherwise nothing more could be done about them. He did not act as if he were representing a friend.

As soon as I left the college, Peter Harris went to see Roger. He confronted him, saying that he had received information regarding convictions, which Roger had not declared on the job application form (the post at the college was not one covered by the Rehabilitation of Offenders Act).

Roger admitted that he had criminal convictions and was asked to tender his resignation. Peter said he could not run the risk of keeping an employee with a criminal background on the staff.

Almost two years later this case surfaced for re-examination, after I had left the health authority and was taking further training in a drug dependency unit.

Roger's solicitor issued a writ for damages, naming the health authority and me. The claim was that, as a result of releasing confidential information, Roger had lost his job and was unable to get another.

The health authority conducted its own investigation and then informed the statutory bodies, thereby calling into question my right to practise.

Thankfully, my detailed records written at the time **99** proved invaluable evidence to support my defence.

Think points

- What factors do you think this CPN could use in defending himself against alleged breach of confidentiality?
- How might you advise a learner nurse to respond when a patient says, 'If I tell you something, promise not to tell anyone?'
- In what instances must client confidentialities be shared?
- Do you think this nurse did break a confidence and breach his position of trust?
- Use this opportunity to acquaint yourself with the recent UKCC document on confidentiality.

The official decision, and discussion

At the UKCC Professional Conduct Committee hearing the allegations were denied. There was no disputing the facts of this case, but the defence hinged on how they were interpreted and the motivation behind the nurse's actions.

For the alleged facts to be proved, the Committee members

had to be satisfied on the following three points – that the information disclosed was confidential; that it had been released without authority or consent; and that the nurse had released it in breach of his position of trust.

On the second point, the nurse's representative argued that instructions from the psychiatrist to prepare a social report provided the necessary consent. This was not upheld in respect of the nurse's role in confidentiality and personal accountability.

After careful consideration, the Committee was satisfied that the information disclosed was confidential and that it had been released without authority or consent.

However, the Committee felt that this nurse had made careful inquiries and had every reason to believe that the person with whom he was sharing the information could be seen as a longstanding close friend, who just happened to have recently become the client's employer.

The nurse had given great consideration to the matter before sharing the information, and could refer back to personal notes to corroborate this. He could not be held to be at fault because the information was misused at a later date.

The Committee suspected that the defendant's friend and employer had always known about the convictions and was willing to turn a blind eye until it emerged that the information was known to others.

Finally, the Committee decided that, rather than having acted in breach of his position of trust, the nurse had sought to honour it. The charge was therefore not proven and the case was closed.

This case showed how community psychiatric nursing services are sometimes set up in a totally inappropriate way. Here was a nurse, appointed to an extremely responsible position, who had limited and irrelevant experience, inadequate resources and unhelpful managers.

Dangerous liaisons

Whenever people mix together there is always the possibility of sexual attraction, even in a caring situation. Indeed, the physical and emotional proximity within nursing can develop into a meaningful relationship, and nurses sometimes marry their patients. Nurses must, however, be aware of the powerful impact of kindness, nurturing and dependency and be careful not to let romantic inclinations compromise professional integrity.

❝❝ At her third attempt Judy Beck was finally appointed sister in the alcoholic unit, working opposite me, the charge nurse. From the outset I thought she was unsuitable; she seemed emotionally vulnerable and unable to distance herself from manipulative characters.

The unit was housed in a redundant villa, separated from the main psychiatric hospital. It was run on therapeutic community principles, and offered a six-week treatment regime.

It was Dr Fielding's project but, with increased demands on him from the acute admission wards, the nurses took on the regular running of our mixed-sex unit. Judy and I led the two teams, arranging to have one trained member of staff on duty around the clock. Being a specialist area, we could expect little help from the main hospital, and hardly ever asked for it. Unit staff altered shifts and rotated internally to ensure cover for sickness, absence and holidays. We were allowed to work in a self contained, autonomous way.

Judy Beck took advantage of this flexibility and I found her altering her duties as she thought fit, irrespective of the needs of the unit. She would hang around in the afternoon or evening and then claim time in lieu to be taken when it suited her. The duty rota rarely reflected her actual presence.

Judy went through periods of being constantly in the unit, when something or someone especially interested her. Her holidays were arranged at inappropriate times, and were often inconvenient for the unit.

We had several rows about her erratic attendance and I spoke once to the area manager to sort things out. Judy continued to be a law unto herself and I despaired of her irregular work pattern.

When Simon Lane was admitted, I predicted trouble. Then I saw in his case notes that Judy had ignored our assessment protocol by admitting him while a court case was pending. I openly confronted Judy and told her to be careful, for I sensed a physical attraction between her and Simon. My remarks angered and embarrassed her but I felt they were necessary.

Later a staff nurse heard Judy criticising me in front of a group of clients, saying that I showed favouritism. This nurse already felt his authority was being undermined by the sister's relaxation of rules. When on night duty, she would allow clients to stay up into the small hours watching videos, making it difficult for the staff nurse to impose the rules when he was in charge.

And Judy had once failed to report for her night duty, without explanation, so the staff nurse had been obliged to rush back to cover the unit.

Within a few weeks Judy's favouritism towards Simon was noticed by other clients. She was attentive to him to the exclusion of others, choosing to sit by him, playing games or talking.

Several clients confided their grievances to the night enrolled nurse, saying they felt they were not getting their share of treatment. Nurse Vickery repeated this but Judy said bluntly that she was intending to have an affair with Simon when he left the unit. His wife and child were no deterrent, as Judy was prepared to take on the child, too.

Nurse Vickery told her she was silly to contemplate such things but Judy just shrugged her shoulders and then glared at the nurse, implying that she should mind her own business. Judy was inclined to change from being friendly, open and frank to someone who would pull rank, as the occasion suited. This produced a rather unpredictable atmosphere for junior staff.

The Thursday evening before Simon was discharged, Judy handed over to Nurse Vickery, who then continued her duties. Judy said she had to see someone and Nurse Vickery presumed they were in the interview room because the light was on. It was not unusual for the sister to remain behind to see a client's relative or friend, or the psychologist.

Nurse Vickery was surprised however, to see Judy coming downstairs from the clients' dormitory area at 1 am, accompanied by Simon, dressed in his pyjamas. Sister made a coffee, which she took to the office, then washed her face and reapplied her make-up, as if preparing to go home.

Suddenly, Judy told the astounded EN that she was going to Simon's room and off she went. Nurse Vickery was at a loss to know what to do at such a late hour; she simply hoped the sister would come back down quickly.

Judy reappeared at five that morning, looking completely dishevelled; she was without make-up and her hair was all over the place. One of her earrings was missing, and she had several 'love-bites' on her neck.

When Nurse Vickery asked about the state Judy was in, she could only reply, 'Oh, what have I done, what have I done?' Judy confessed that she'd had sex with Simon, but this was not the first time.

The previous Monday she had volunteered to use some time

owing to cover for Nurse Vickery's night off, and had sex with Simon then. Apparently, the affair had started on the day of Simon's assessment, before his admission, just as I had suspected.

Judy's main concern was the three love-bites above her collar and she asked Nurse Vickery whether she should cover them with plasters. Judy's jewellery was missing – a locket, rings and a watch. She explained that they were on Simon's dressing table.

At 6 am, Judy's husband rang but Nurse Vickery could not hear any of their conversation. Just then another client came downstairs. Judy told the enrolled nurse to explain that she had come on duty in order to let the night nurse go early.

The client retorted indignantly, 'Oh, don't be ridiculous, we aren't blind – and we aren't deaf either!'

It was obvious that the clients were fully aware of the night's events by the time Nurse Vickery left duty at 7 am.

The assistant nurse arrived on day duty to be met by an unkempt, weary and preoccupied sister. Remarking on her appearance, the assistant nurse was told of the affair with Simon and how Judy had spent most of the night with him.

Judy was adamant that the relationship would continue after his discharge and was obviously besotted with Simon. Sister, the assistant nurse, and a student continued with the morning work. At coffee time, Judy admitted to the assistant that she had been a fool and now saw the error of her ways.

She was not talking about the error of professional indiscretion but the error of tearing up the telephone number she had given to Simon before he left the unit. It appeared that what was worrying Judy was that there might be some difficulty in continuing their relationship.

She wrote to Simon on a piece of hospital notepaper, with the pretext of telling him about a local workshop on alcoholism. She included her own telephone number but signed the letter with the assistant's name. When the assistant protested, Judy tore up that letter, then sent a scrappy note to Simon with the ward phone number, asking him to ring her.

Judy was due to hand over to me at 1.30 pm, when I would be returning from a week's leave, and finish her shift at 2 pm. However, she went home just after 11 am, complaining of feeling upset and not wanting to face the charge nurse. She left an assistant nurse in charge of the unit, a student running group therapy and the drug keys unsupervised in the office drawer.

She did not report her absence to anyone in authority, and all this was contrary to hospital policy. When I came on duty, I was greeted by the now public knowledge of the previous night's events.

Judy Beck was sacked and called before a hearing of the UKCC Professional Conduct Committee, which she did not attend.

156

The police were not involved. It is not an offence under the Mental Health Act for a female staff member to have sex with a male client. However, similar activity by a male or female nurse would be seen as equally un-

99

acceptable in professional terms.

Think points

- There are a number of areas of weakness in professional conduct by this nurse; identify them.
- There are various occasions when personal gain outweighs professional responsibility. Name any you know of.
- In the setting of an alcohol treatment centre, what particular difficulties might be encountered regarding interpersonal relationships?
- How might you counsel or advise a junior member of staff who fears a strong personal involvement with a patient or client?
- Do you think this nurse should lose her right to practise?

The official decision, and discussion

It was surprising that this fairly intense psychotherapy unit was devoid of staff support, providing no forum to thrash out difficulties or challenge performance.

Management appeared content to allow the unit to function with clinical autonomy, intervening as troubleshooters only when asked to help, but failing to make any follow-up review.

There were obvious tensions between the team leaders, together with some questionable behaviour by the sister. Other staff were left to absorb problems, feeling frustrated and powerless when confronted by unprofessional practices which challenged their loyalties. Unfortunately, the sister's earlier misdemeanours went unchecked and she appeared to have little personal control or professional conscience. Nor was there managerial influence to curtail her activities.

The sister faced a number of allegations related to her practice but was found guilty on the major charges of having an unprofessional relationship, and sexual intercourse with a patient. Her name was removed from the UKCC Register.

Useful addresses

UKCC – United Kingdom Central Council for Nursing, Midwifery
      and Health Visiting
23 Portland Place
London W1N 3AF   Tel: 071–637 7181

ENB – English National Board
Victory House
170 Tottenham Court Road
London W1P 0HA   Tel: 071–388 3131

WNB – Welsh National Board
13th Floor, Pearl Assurance House
Greyfriars Road
Cardiff CF1 3RT   Tel: 0222–395535

NBS – National Board for Scotland
22 Queen Street
Edinburgh EH2 1JX   Tel: 031–226 7371

NBNI – National Board for Northern Ireland
RAC House
79 Chichester Street
Belfast BT1 4JE   Tel: 0232–238152

NWS – Nurses' Welfare Service
Victoria Chambers
16/18 Strutton Ground
London SW1P 2HP   Tel: 071–222 1563/4

RCN – Royal College of Nursing
20 Cavendish Square
London W1M 0AB   Tel: 071–409 3333